BURNS AND SCALDS
86/87 — Swift emergency action with burns and scalds – among the most common of household injuries. The treatment of minor injuries at home and priority action for more serious cases.

POISONS AND CORROSIVES
88/89 — One of the most urgent of all emergencies, particularly if the victim is a young child. Action priorities to be followed.

SHOCK AND FAINTING
90/91 — Causes of shock and fainting. When, and when not, to call for urgent medical attention. The treatment of shock in the home.

EMERGENCY CHILDBIRTH
92/93 — Not the most common household emergency – but one for which everyone should be prepared.

EYE INJURIES AND SPLINTERS
94/95 — Fast relief from what are usually minor, inconvenient, injuries. Emergency measures to be adopted in cases of serious injury.

BITES AND STINGS
96/97 — One of the most common outdoor hazards. Immediate action to relieve pain and inflammation, and avoid infection. Emergency action for serious cases.

Emergency Telephone Numbers

Ambulance	_____
Fire Department	_____
Police Department	_____
Taxi	_____
Family doctor	
office	_____
home	_____
Hospital emergency ward	_____
maternity ward	_____
Poison Control Center	_____
Dentist	_____
Pharmacist	_____
Coastguard	_____
Nearest relative	_____
Nearest neighbor	_____

CONSULTANTS: DR. TONY SMITH qualified as a physician in 1959 and, following a series of hospital appointments in England, became a full-time medical journalist in 1965. He is currently Deputy Editor of the *British Medical Journal* and the medical correspondent of the London *Times*. **DR. RICHARD V. LEE**, a graduate of Yale University School of Medicine, is currently Chief of the Medical Service at the Buffalo Veterans Administration Hospital in Buffalo, New York, and Professor of Medicine and Vice Chairman of the Department of Internal Medicine at the State University of New York.

CONSULTING EDITOR: BILL BRECKON is a widely respected British author, journalist, and broadcaster specializing in medical and scientific affairs. He has written several books and has worked extensively on radio and television educational programs.

CONTRIBUTORS: SUE COOK has worked in book publishing and is currently co-presenter of the BBC magazine program, 'You and Yours.' **NICK LANDON** is Executive Editor of *Pulse*, the newspaper of the British medical profession and is also the Deputy Chairman of the Medical Journalists' Association in London.

ACCIDENT ACTION

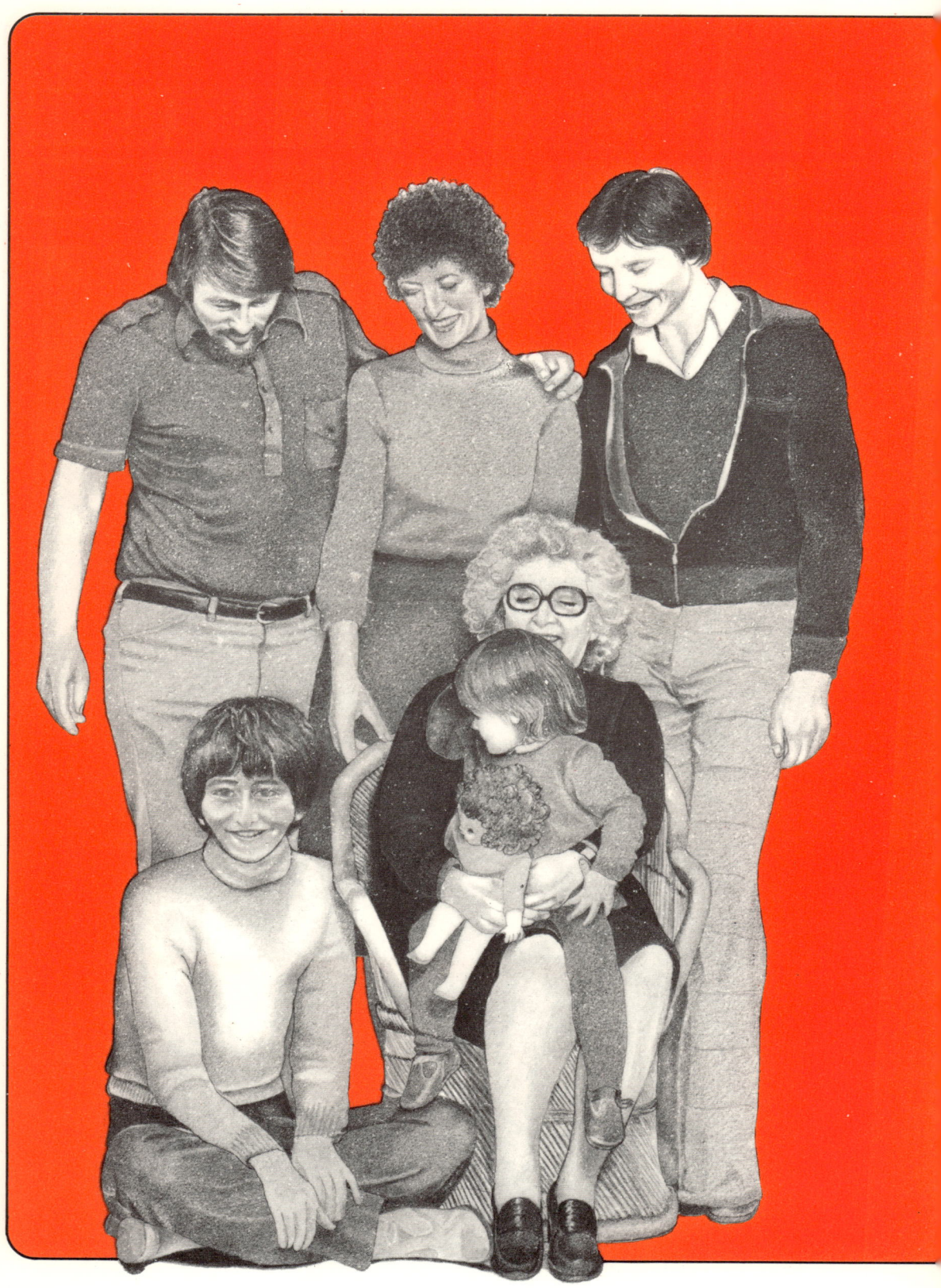

THE ESSENTIAL FAMILY GUIDE TO HOME SAFETY AND FIRST AID

ACCIDENT ACTION

A STUDIO BOOK
THE VIKING PRESS · NEW YORK

Accident Action was conceived, edited and designed by Harrow House Editions Limited, 104, High Street, Harrow-on-the-Hill, Middlesex HA1 3LP, England.

Copyright © Harrow House Editions Ltd. 1978
All rights reserved.

Published in 1979 by The Viking Press
625 Madison Avenue, New York, N.Y. 10022

Published simultaneously in Canada by
Penguin Books Canada Limited

Typeset in Century Schoolbook by
Woolaston Parker Ltd. Leicester, England.
Illustrations originated by
Photoprint Plates Ltd. Rayleigh, England.
Printed and bound by
Dai Nippon, Hong Kong.

Library of Congress Cataloging in Publication Data
Main entry under title:
   Accident action.
   (A Studio book)
   Includes index.
   1. First aid in illness and injury.   2. Home accidents.   I. Breckon, William.

RC86.7.A25   614.8'53   78-10670
ISBN 0-670-10206-7

Consultants: Dr Richard V. Lee, United States
Dr Tony Smith, England

Consultant Editor: Bill Breckon

Contributors: Sue Cook
Nick Landon

Contents

10-11	The Aims of First Aid	66-67	Bleeding: Foot, Knee and Elbow
12-13	The Family	68-69	Bleeding: Finger and Head
14-15	Safety in the Home	70-71	Loss of Consciousness
		72-73	Broken Bones: Arm, Hand and Elbow
	THE FAMILY AND HOME		
16-17	Mother	74-75	Broken Bones: Lower Leg and Thigh
18-19	Father		
20-21	Three-year-old	76-77	Broken Bones: Knee and Foot
22-23	Ten-year-old		
24-25	Teenager	78-79	Broken Bones: Spine and Pelvis
26-27	Grandparent		
28-29	Kitchen	80-81	Broken Bones: Collarbone and Ribs
30-31	Bathroom		
32-33	Bedroom and Stairs	82-83	Broken Bones: Jaw and Skull
34-35	Living room		
36-37	Garage and Workshop	84-85	Sprain, Strain and Dislocation
38-39	Garden	86-87	Burns and Scalds
40-41	Toxic Plants	88-89	Poisons and Corrosives
42-43	The First Aid Kit	90-91	Shock and Fainting
44-45	Home Cures	92-93	Emergency Childbirth
46-47	The Fire Risk	94-95	Splinters and Eye Injuries
		96-97	Bites and Stings
48-49	ACCIDENT ACTION Action Priorities	98-99	GOING AWAY Vacation Preparations
50-51	Breathing Stopped		
52-53	Artificial Respiration: The 'Kiss of Life'	100-101	Automobile Accidents
		102-103	Outdoor Life
54-55	Artificial Respiration: Holger-Nielsen Method	104-105	Hiking and Spelunking
		106-107	Sun and Heat
56-57	Sylvester Method	108-109	Water Sports
58-59	Heart Stopped	110-111	Winter Sports
60-61	Heart Attack	112-113	Shooting, Racquet Sports and Jogging
62-63	Bleeding: Types of Wound		
64-65	Bleeding: Arm and Hand	114-117	Index and Credits

The Aims of First Aid

Although sensible precautions will greatly minimize the risk, accidents can happen to anyone, anywhere and at any time. Prompt action based on a working knowledge of first aid will reduce the effect of an injury, speed recovery and, in extreme cases, save the casualty's life. Remember that the life you save could well be that of a member of your own family for most accidents occur in the home or while the family is out together.

The best way to learn first aid is to attend a course run by one of the established first aid training organizations, such as the Red Cross, where you will receive instruction and the opportunity to practice under the guidance of an experienced first aider. However, you can learn the basic techniques from books – in which case involve as many as possible of your family and friends.

It is very important to remember that first aid is just that: *first* aid. It is not full and complete treatment but essential action designed to minimize the effect of the injury and stabilize the casualty's condition until experts can take over.

The circumstances of each accident will be different and the first aider will have to adapt his approach accordingly – sometimes even breaking some of the 'rules' if common sense and circumstance require it. The following is a flexible, rational plan of action suitable, with some modification, for most accident situations:

- ☐ *Keep calm, take charge, organize:* enlist the help of bystanders immediately, sending for ambulance and other emergency services; keeping back crowds; controlling traffic; keeping people clear of hazards such as spilt corrosives or live electrical equipment.
- ☐ *Withdraw from danger:* if danger still threatens from fire, leaking gas or toxic liquids, get yourself and the casualty away from danger as quickly as possible. However if there is no immediate further danger, examine and treat the casualty where he is. Do not attempt to move him until you know the extent of his injuries.
- ☐ *Begin first aid:* quickly check the following points and take immediate action;

> BREATHING: If respiration is weak or stopped, give artificial respiration.
> CHOKING: Clear the casualty's airway. Many accident victims die simply from blockage of the airways.
> BLEEDING: Control severe bleeding promptly and note any evidence of internal injury.
> UNCONSCIOUSNESS: Ensure that the airways are clear and place the casualty in the recovery position, but check first for injury to neck or spine.

Keep talking to the casualty, he will be frightened and confused. Reassure him and tell him what you are doing. If you have to leave him to attend to a more seriously injured person, explain this to him.

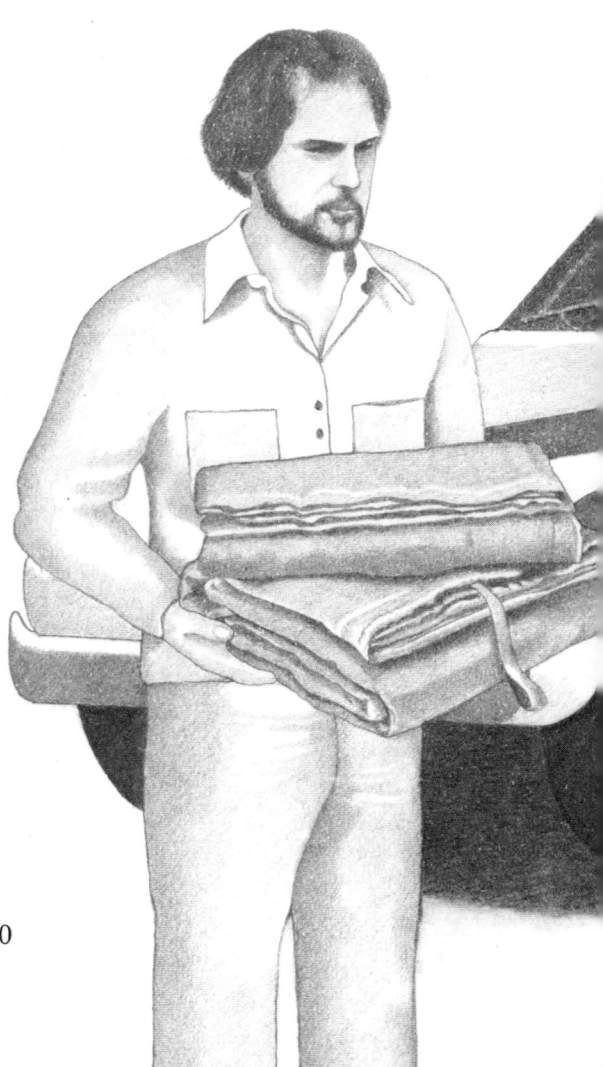

Be methodical. Having taken action on any immediate threats to life, begin a thorough examination for other wounds and broken bones. If the casualty is conscious, ask him about his injuries. He may later lose consciousness, or become confused, and the more information you can pass on to the emergency services, the better. Improvise where necessary and don't try to be sophisticated; remember this is *first* aid. Do not give anything by mouth except to moisten the lips of a conscious burned casualty. Treat major injuries, keep casualties warm, calm and reassured, and summon help quickly.

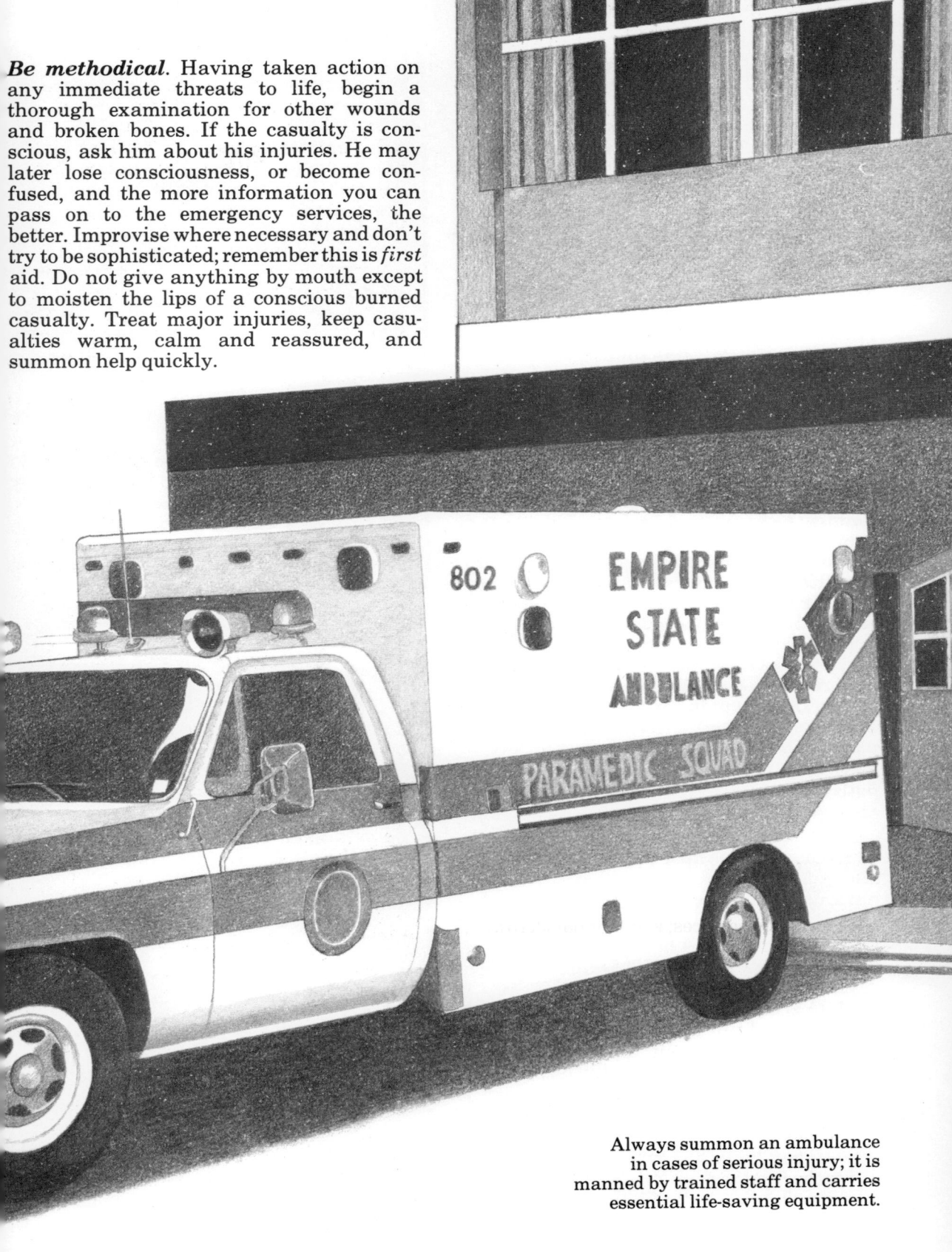

Always summon an ambulance in cases of serious injury; it is manned by trained staff and carries essential life-saving equipment.

The Family

It is a very common failing to think that accidents happen only to other people. Alas nothing could be further from the truth: nobody is completely isolated from risk. Nevertheless, if you are aware of everyday hazards and take common sense precations, the risks can be greatly reduced.

Of course the pattern of risk is not the same for every member of the family. Some groups, particularly the young, the elderly and the physically or mentally handicapped, are more prone to accidents than others.

Home accidents in Europe account for between 1 and 2 percent of all deaths and for each fatal accident there are probably about 150 non-fatal home accidents requiring hospital treatment or prolonged home care.

In the United States, for example, about 16 million people are injured every year in or around the home, and between 700,000 and 1 million of these are estimated to result from toys or other children's products. In western countries, the major causes of injury include falls, fires, burns and scalds, electrocution, suffocation and poisoning.

The infant is most at risk from falls, cuts and bruises and poisoning but the vast majority of deaths due to 'mechanical suffocation' occur in children under five, and are frequently due to the child having pulled a plastic bag over his head.

Between the ages of five and fourteen, the pattern changes and cuts, bruises and occasional breaks become more common.

Alcohol, smoking, motor vehicle accidents and injuries incurred in various sports and outdoor leisure activities are the major hazards facing the teenager, while for the parents, everyday household activities such as cooking, lifting, household maintenance and gardening are the cause of the majority of injuries requiring medical treatment.

Among the elderly, the slowing down of reactions and the almost inevitable deterioration of the senses, leads to more falls, burns and scalds, and to an increased risk of accidental overdose or gassing.

Put this way, it sounds as though anyone living to a ripe old age must bear a charmed life – but simple precautions and a basic knowledge of first aid will ensure that most homes remain free of major accidents.

A recent survey showed that approximately one person in 53 was disabled for one or more days by injuries suffered in home accidents. About 10,000 injuries resulted in some permanent impairment. The total number of deaths from home accidents was around 25,500 in one single year.

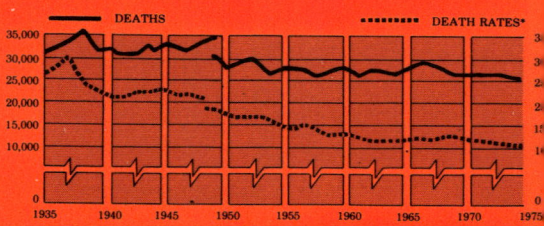

*Per 10,000 population adjusted to the age distribution of the population in 1940

Accidental deaths and death rates
Deaths in 1975 were about the same as in 1935, allowing for the 1948 classification changes. Today, however, there are many more people in the susceptible over 65 and under 5 age groups.

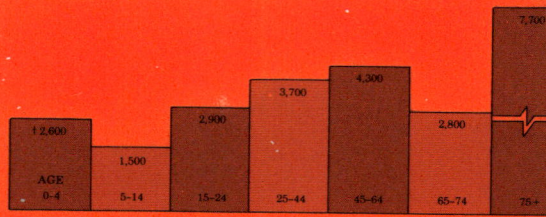

† Number of deaths

Fatal accidents (all causes)
Includes deaths in the home and on home premises to occupants, guests, trespassers and domestic employees.

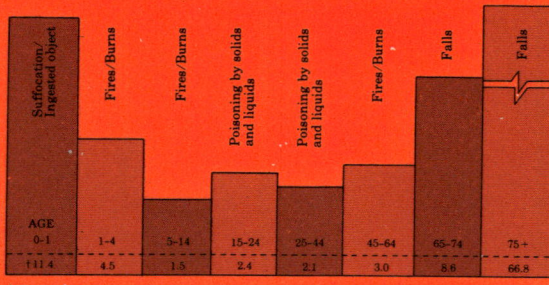

† Deaths per 100,000 population in each age group

Accident type by age group
The principal type of accident in each age group in one year indicates that, in those over 65 years, falling is the most common cause of death.

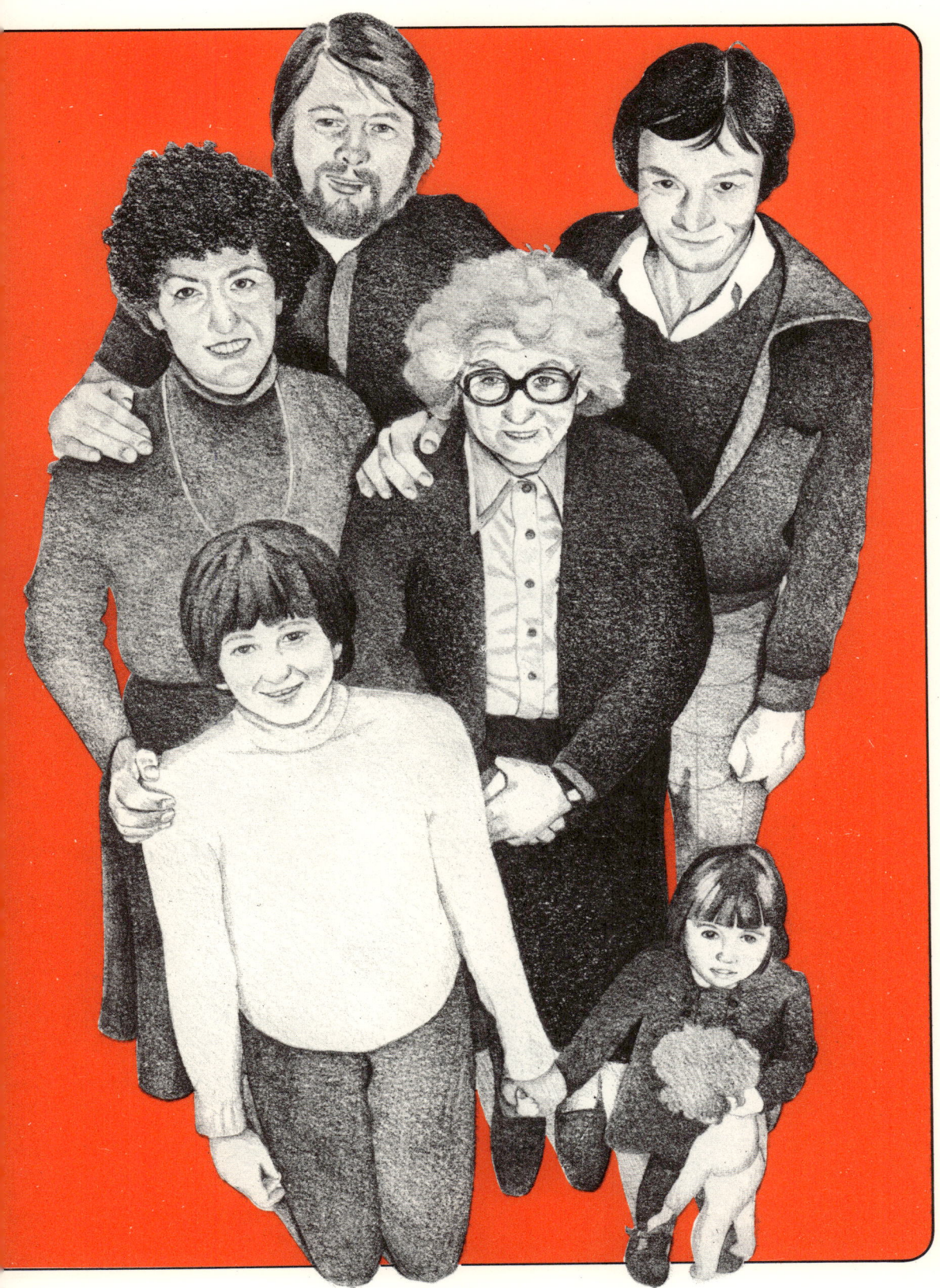

Safety in the Home

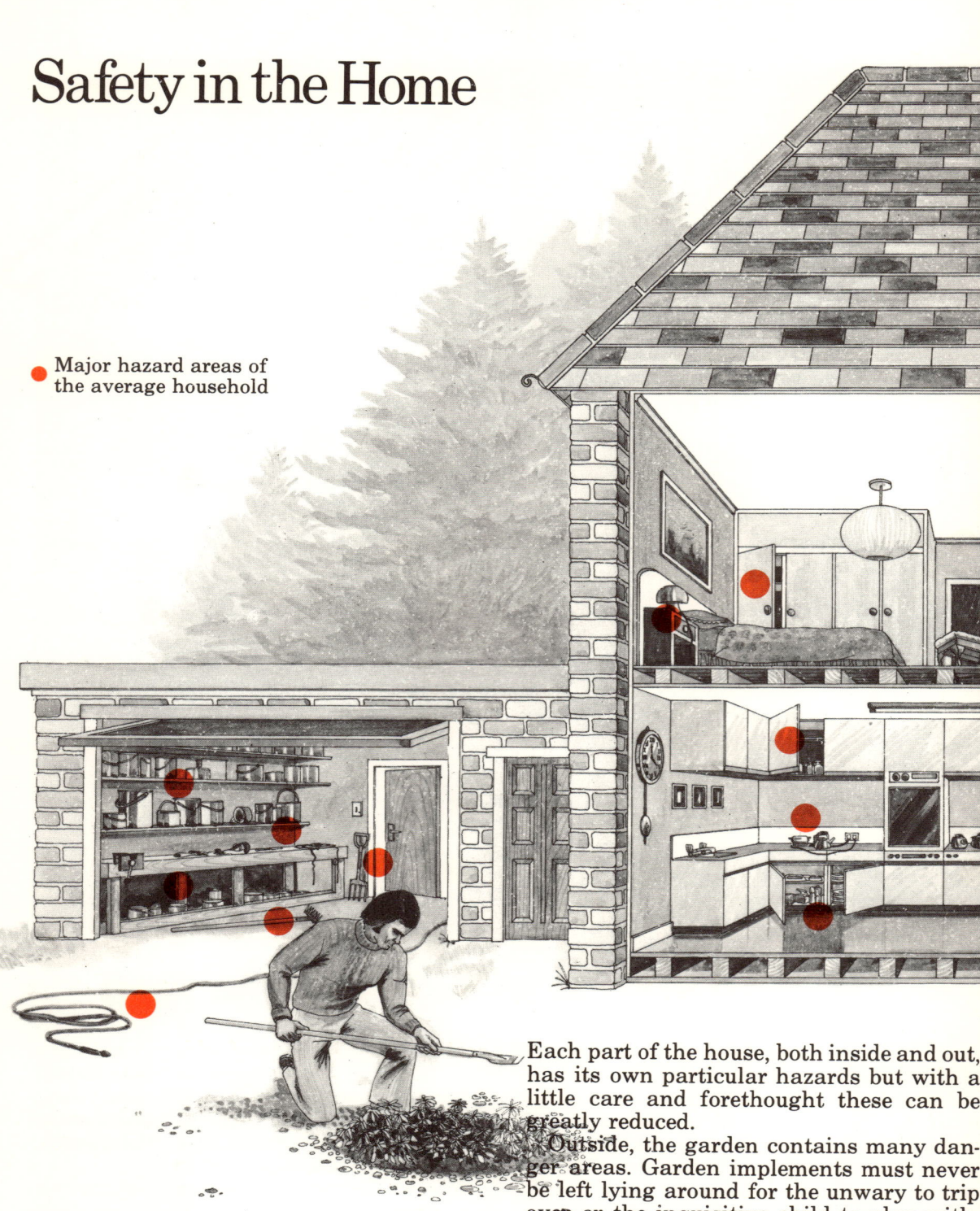

● Major hazard areas of the average household

Each part of the house, both inside and out, has its own particular hazards but with a little care and forethought these can be greatly reduced.

Outside, the garden contains many danger areas. Garden implements must never be left lying around for the unwary to trip over or the inquisitive child to play with. Power tools such as hedge trimmers or mowers are particularly dangerous in the wrong hands. Fertilizers, herbicides and pesticides, like all other dangerous chemicals, should only be stored in clearly-marked

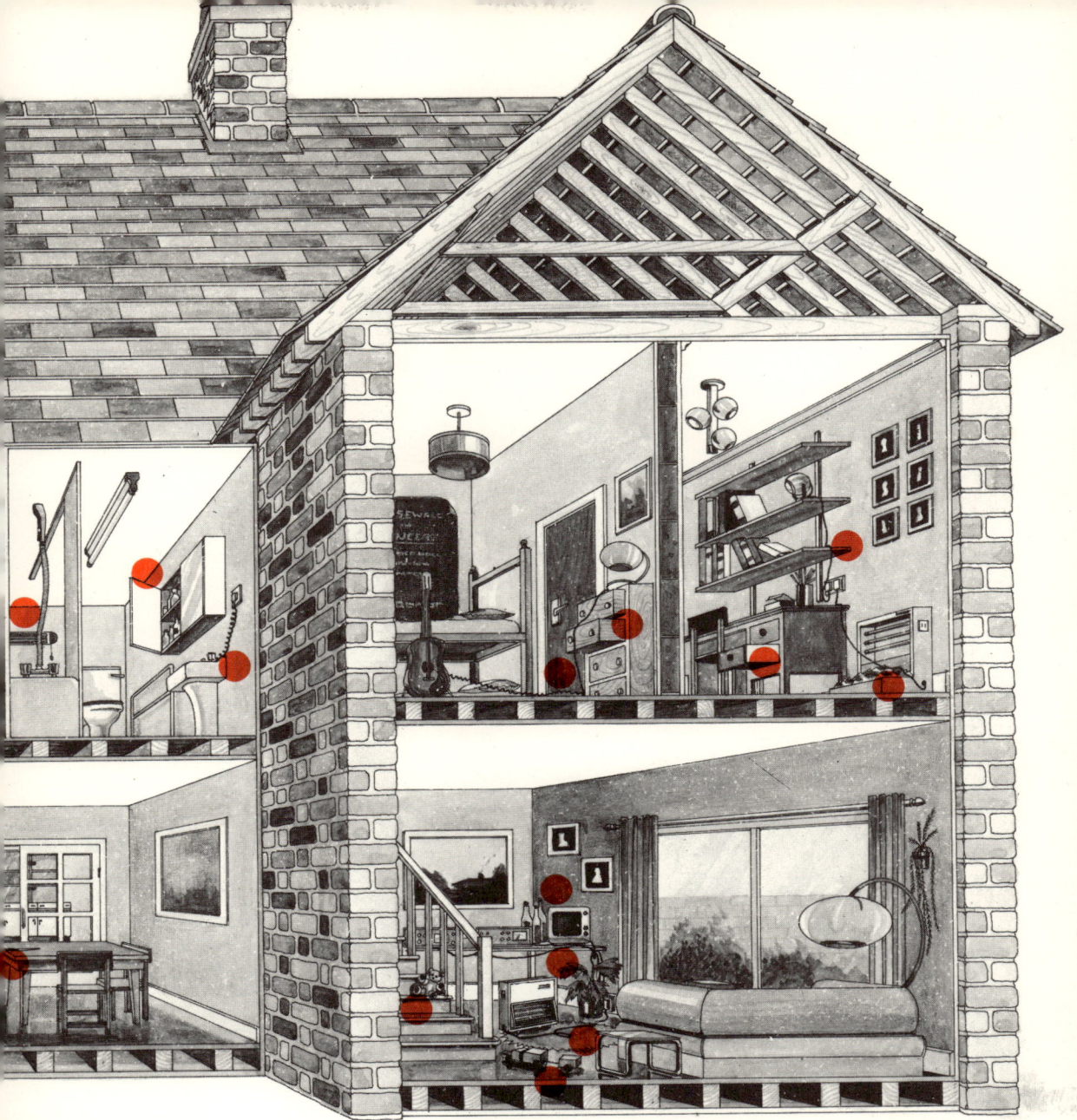

containers, and even then well out of reach of children.

Around the house, all paths and steps must be maintained in good repair and should, wherever possible, be well lit. Ornamental ponds may look attractive but constitute a serious hazard to very small children; they should be fenced off, or better still drained until the children are older.

Safety within the home is largely a matter of common sense - and yet thousands of men, women and children every year require hospital treatment for falls, cuts, burns and scalds - the majority of which could have been avoided. All sharp implements should be kept in drawers, particularly when young children are about, and all medications should be stored well out of a child's reach, preferably in a locked cabinet.

Faulty electrical wiring, and equipment, constitute a grave danger - and a constant fire hazard. Check all systems regularly and take expert advice if in doubt. Cutting corners, leaving damage unrepaired or lighting and heating systems without proper maintenance, is simply asking for trouble.

Mother

Although more and more 'labor-saving' items are being made available to the mother and housewife, these could by no means be described as 'accident-preventing'. Indeed, the mother is probably exposed to more potential accidents than any other member of the family.

However simple the can opener may be to operate, the resultant jagged edge is just as sharp and liable to cut. However simple to operate may be the burner, the hot fat is just as liable to spit. However easy the polish may be to apply, the floor ends up just as slippery.

Many of the most obvious hazards can be found in the KITCHEN (SEE **pp. 28-9**). Burns or scalds from pans on the burner or from the kettle; cuts from kitchen knives or other implements, from the edges of open cans or from broken glass or china ware; electric shock from any of the varied domestic appliances such as knife sharpeners, mixers, and so on.

Simple safety measures

A few sensible precautions can make accidents far less likely. To avoid cuts, never continue to use chipped or cracked glass or china, remembering also that the cracks can harbor the organisms causing food poisoning. Care in the use of sharp kitchen implements is essential, however much the haste, and the same applies to opened cans.

If there is cooking on the stove, keep pan handles turned *inwards* so that they do not

When preparing vegetables or meat use a firm base, a sharp knife, and pay attention.

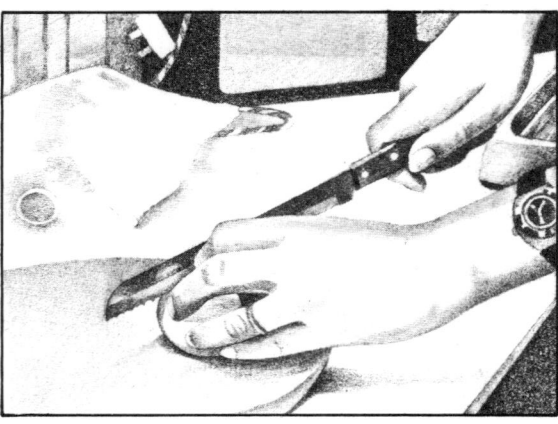

protrude over the edge where they may catch on clothing and spill. In the event of a fire in the frying pan, on no account try to dowse it with water; this will cause the hot fat to spit and flare violently, shooting burning droplets in all directions.

In all rooms, use a non-slip polish and see that all loose mats have at least a strip of non-slip backing.

A small domestic fire extinguisher near the cooker is a good idea, particularly as this can be chosen so that it will quench electrical fires with safety **(see pp 46-7)**.

Never attempt to connect domestic appliances and do not attempt to change the plugs with which they come equipped. Never continue to use any appliance which has bare wires exposed or a cable covering that is frayed, scorched or otherwise damaged. Make sure that cables cannot touch any part of the stove top or oven.

In November 1977 a horrifying report was published in Britain revealing that of the 400 million plugs estimated to be in daily use, more than 73 million could be in a dangerous condition through inefficient cord grips; another 12 million through physical damage to the body of the plug, and more than six million through incorrect wiring. The message is quite clear. Do not use a plug if you suspect faulty wiring or if the plug is chipped or broken. Call an electrician if in any doubt.

Take special care on stairs. Never carry such a heavy load that you might lose your balance – it is far better to make two trips and be safe.
Indeed, never lift a load which is too heavy for you. When you *do* lift, don't bend forward so that the strain is all taken by the back – at the risk of a slipped disk or torn muscle. Rather, keep a straight back and bend your knees.

When you are dusting awkward corners high in the room, make sure that you are standing on something stable that won't wobble or topple over. It is better to use the household steps than to improvise.

If you rely on portable heaters – oil or electric – for warmth, keep well away from them when, for instance, you are folding a tablecloth, in case you cause a fire. *Never* move an oil heater when it is burning. If at all possible heaters should be secured to the wall so that they cannot be knocked over.

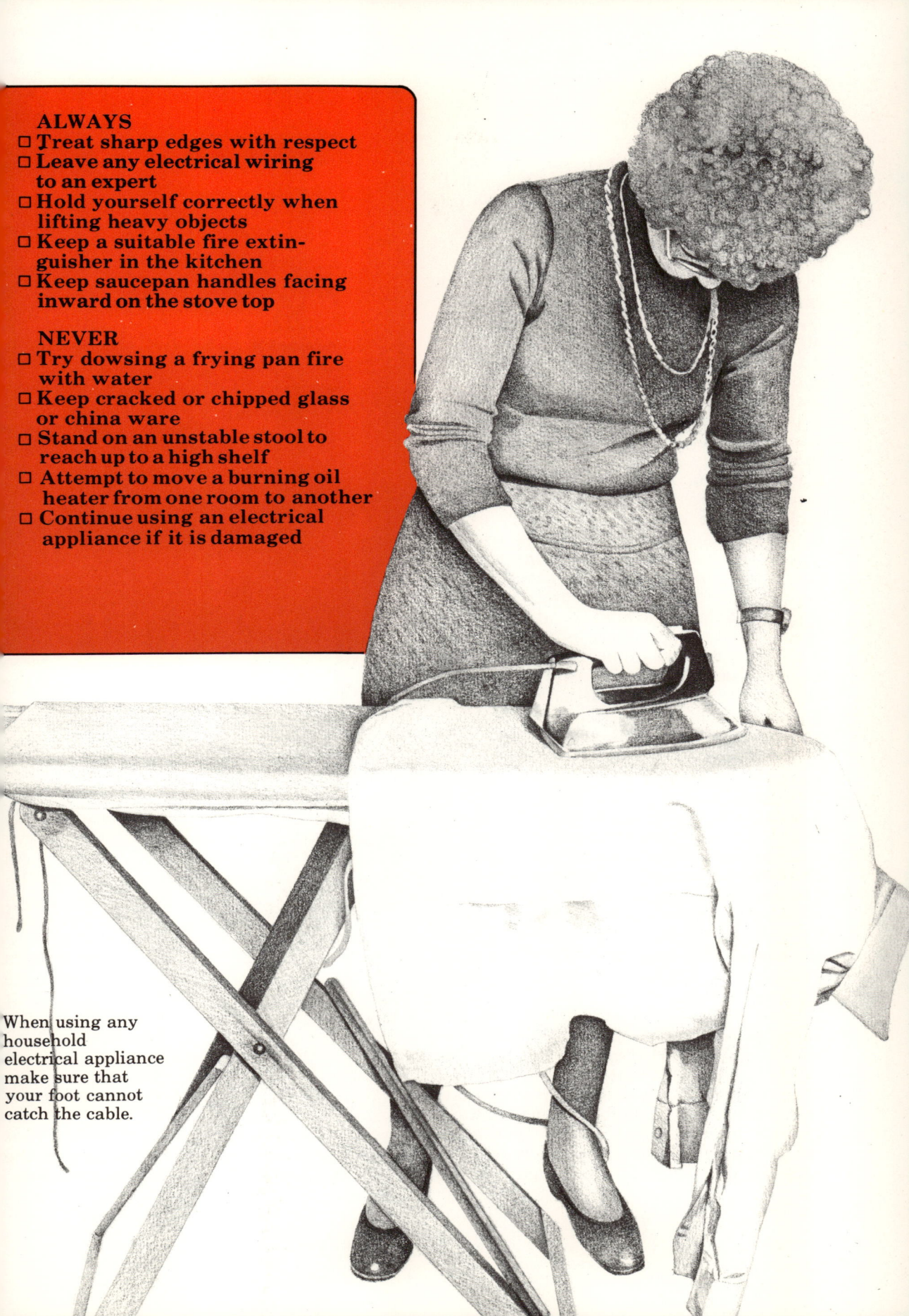

ALWAYS
- Treat sharp edges with respect
- Leave any electrical wiring to an expert
- Hold yourself correctly when lifting heavy objects
- Keep a suitable fire extinguisher in the kitchen
- Keep saucepan handles facing inward on the stove top

NEVER
- Try dowsing a frying pan fire with water
- Keep cracked or chipped glass or china ware
- Stand on an unstable stool to reach up to a high shelf
- Attempt to move a burning oil heater from one room to another
- Continue using an electrical appliance if it is damaged

When using any household electrical appliance make sure that your foot cannot catch the cable.

Father

In these days of do-it-yourself, the man of the house is liable to turn his hand to innumerable jobs that used to be the preserve of experts, from house repairs to electrical wiring. There is also an urge to 'get fit' in middle age, when he should have kept fit all the time. In all these activities, a little care may prevent harm.

A lot of risk in the home stems from attempts at improvisation. Ladders without a firm footing, or which are not quite long enough; the wrong tool that 'might just do' for the job; the car held above the ground on a pile of bricks so that father can better crawl beneath. These are typical hazards that are easily avoided.

When using tools for wood or metal working of any description, use the correct tool and use it correctly. Beware of the slipping screwdriver, the incorrectly held chisel, the carelessly used hedge trimmer that severs its own cable, the saw that slips because the wood is not securely held.

If you do make a mistake and cause an injury, such as a puncture by a screwdriver, a cut from a sharp implement, an abrasion from the sander on your power tool, *always* cleanse the wound and dress it. It may be tempting to wait until you have finished the job, but you run the risk of serious infection at the wound site.

Keeping fit
Father is also, of course, at risk from the health hazards that are given emphasis by our way of life. Smoking increases the chances of cancer, bronchitis and heart disease, while many men take too little exercise during their normal life and thus need to make a conscious effort to achieve the fitness that may save them from premature ageing, a shorter life due to obesity, or even death from a heart attack.

The art of exercise is, however, not suddenly to decide that it's time for strenuous, violent games, for that way lies potential injury to untrained muscles, back trouble or even a heart attack. If you have not taken regular exercise throughout your adult life, then it is better by far to begin again comparatively gently, slowly increasing the intensity of effort as fitness is regained. Aim

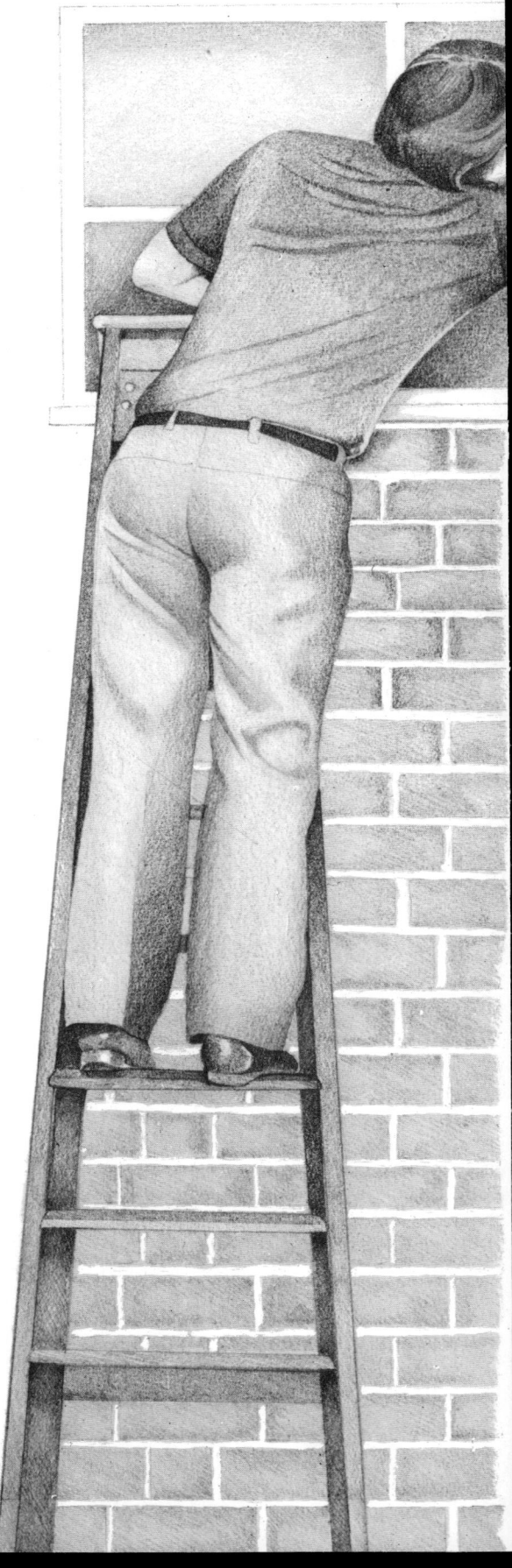

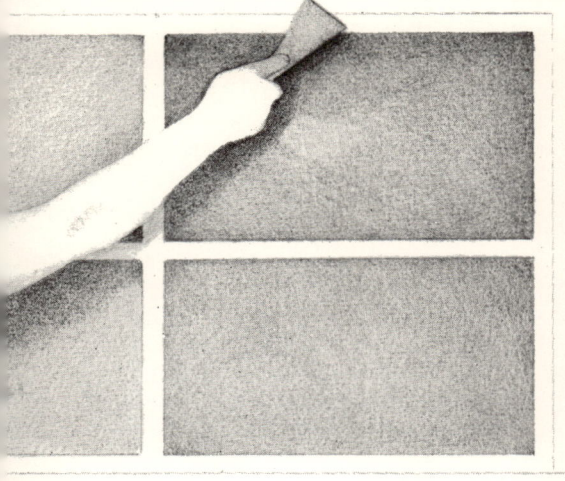

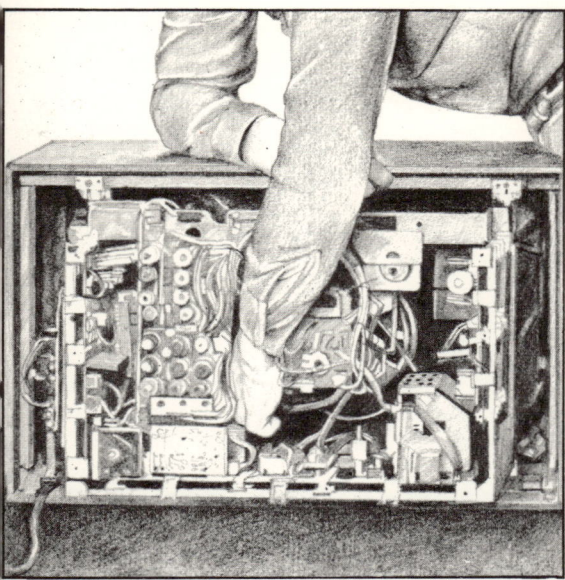

Never remove the back of the television set, even if it is unplugged. A high voltage charge may remain in some of the components.

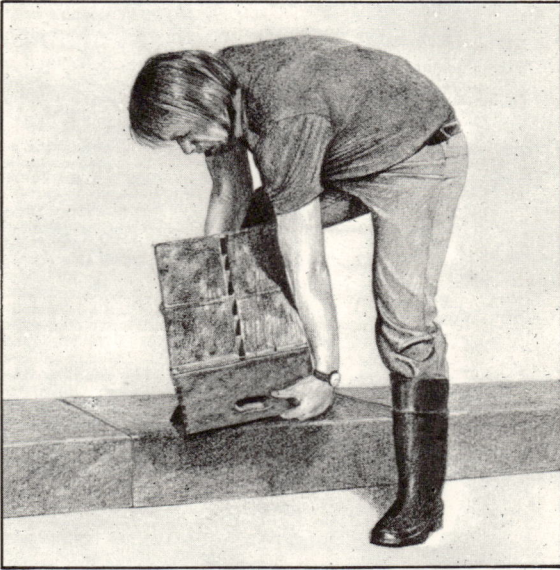

Courting back injury. When lifting heavy objects keep the back as upright as possible; bend the knees and use the leg muscles.

ALWAYS
- ☐ Plan each job carefully
- ☐ Use the right tools for the job
- ☐ Beware of all cutting edges
- ☐ Use leg muscles when lifting

DO NOT
- ☐ Smoke (if you must, cut down)
- ☐ Eat or drink to excess
- ☐ Leave any wound untreated
- ☐ Attempt any electrical wiring unless you are trained
- ☐ Take risks on steps or ladders

eventually to be able to take enough strenuous exercise at least twice a week to raise your pulse rate from its normal 70–80 beats a minute to 120 or more.

Don't undertake violent exercise unless you are already fit. After a winter of inactivity, don't rush out and try to dig the entire garden in one day, or suddenly decide to take up tennis again when you are carrying too much weight after 20 years away from active sport.

Men under the age of 50 are far more likely than women in the same age group to suffer a HEART ATTACK (ACTION DETAILS pp 60-61). Regular exercise (for instance jogging), and limitation of animal fats in the diet, will help to decrease this risk.

It is also worth remembering that too much food or alcohol adds to the health hazards of the middle-aged man. In earlier life the body is more resilient and often seems able to take abuse without lasting damage. Unfortunately this is not the case in the middle and later years.

Three-year-old

At the age of three, a child begins to move away from his earlier total dependence on mother and father. This means that the age of experiment has begun in earnest and, as the three-year-old is quite uncritical, potential dangers must be foreseen by parents if accidents are to be prevented.

The three-year-old will still spend a lot of time following his parents around the home, so extra care must be taken whenever the parent is performing some potentially dangerous task. However, the same child can disappear as if by magic, to get into trouble elsewhere if hazards are left unguarded.

The household danger zones
In the kitchen, for instance, all sharp utensils and knives should be kept in a drawer where the curious toddler cannot get hold of them. Saucepan handles should *never* be allowed to protrude over the side of the stove, in case little hands drag them off and cause scalds. Cleaning materials and, particularly, bleach and disinfectants, must be kept in a cupboard, preferably locked.

In the living room, fires must be adequately guarded by screens that cannot be pulled away by the child.

Stairs are always a hazard, for in many countries falls are the most common cause of injury to children requiring medical treatment. See that lighting is good, and ensure that toys are not left lying about for children to trip over.

In the bedroom, windows must either be secured or fitted with protective-mesh screens or bars. Heaters, electric fans and air conditioning units *must* be electrically safe and regularly maintained.

In the bathroom, all drugs, medicines and pills *must* be kept in a cabinet out of reach of the small child, and preferably locked.

Out in the garden, the sandbox should not be deep enough for a child to be buried, and ponds should be fenced off even though they may only be shallow. Keep garden tools such as rakes and forks out of the way and take particular care that your three-year-old is not anywhere nearby when outdoor power tools such as mowers or hedge trimmers are in use.

Small children are one of the most accident-prone groups of people, but common sense can avoid many hazards. Typically, remember to keep all plastic bags out of the way so that the child cannot put them over his head and suffocate – and beware of small foreign bodies such as (metal) nuts, for the child may experiment and force them into his nose or ear.

Finally, although nobody would condemn the habit of keeping a family pet, remember that cats or dogs can be disease carriers, so make sure that the child always washes his hands after playing with the pet.

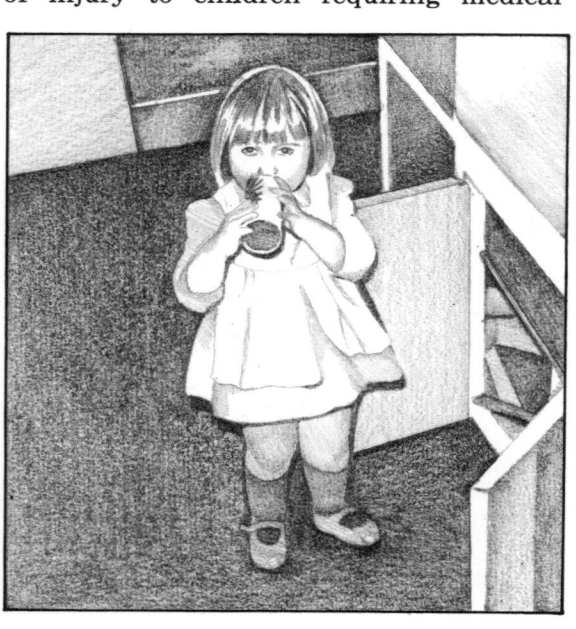
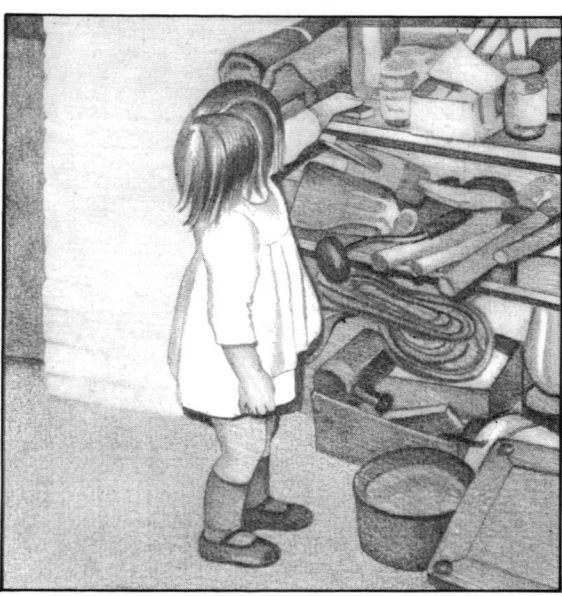

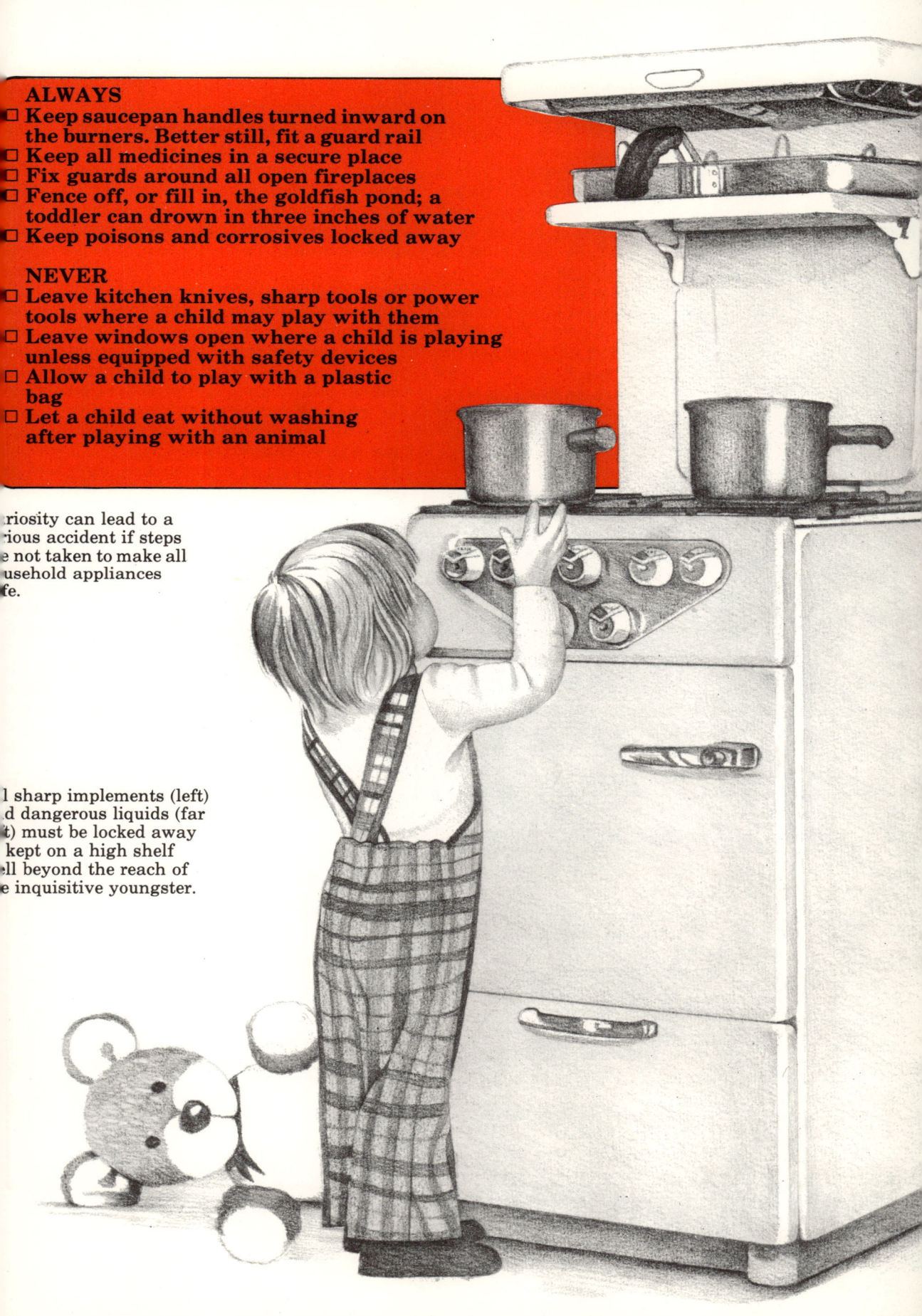

ALWAYS
- ☐ Keep saucepan handles turned inward on the burners. Better still, fit a guard rail
- ☐ Keep all medicines in a secure place
- ☐ Fix guards around all open fireplaces
- ☐ Fence off, or fill in, the goldfish pond; a toddler can drown in three inches of water
- ☐ Keep poisons and corrosives locked away

NEVER
- ☐ Leave kitchen knives, sharp tools or power tools where a child may play with them
- ☐ Leave windows open where a child is playing unless equipped with safety devices
- ☐ Allow a child to play with a plastic bag
- ☐ Let a child eat without washing after playing with an animal

...riosity can lead to a ...ious accident if steps ...e not taken to make all ...usehold appliances ...fe.

...l sharp implements (left) ...d dangerous liquids (far ...t) must be locked away ...kept on a high shelf ...ll beyond the reach of ...e inquisitive youngster.

Ten-year-old

At the age of ten, children often feel that they are no longer one of the 'little kids'. It is not that they feel they are yet one of the big ones – but they begin to look ahead to the time when they will be. Nevertheless, they are still likely at times to lapse into babyish behavior, so you can't altogether relax the safety rules applying to small children.

Of course, the ten-year-old is fast becoming more active and more mobile. You will be less likely to find him or her falling down the stairs because the balance is far more certain, but activities such as tree-climbing, roller skating, cycling, skateboarding and so on are all potentially dangerous.

The age of adventure

You cannot – and should not – try to cocoon your child so that danger is never encountered. It is far better to encourage the child to take his or her own safety precautions such as proper protective clothing and headgear for the skateboarder, and a machine of the right size with properly adjusted saddle and good brakes for the cyclist. You must also be prepared for the almost inevitable accidents.

Cuts, grazes and bruises will be the most common injuries, together with wood splinters which should be removed immediately to avoid infection. Ordinary home first-aid measures will be adequate for most of these, but if a cut looks long and deep, it is as well to check with a doctor that stitches are not needed and if any wound seems to be infected, so that it is not healing, medical attention should be sought.

Luckily, at this age bones are still somewhat 'elastic', so that many falls which would result in fractures in older people will not cause serious damage to the ten-year-old, while others will only cause cracked bones (green-stick fractures) rather than proper breaks. Nevertheless, if you suspect that there is any possibility of a broken bone, seek the doctor's opinion.

On rare occasions, falling from a tree, for instance, may cause internal injuries. Lasting and severe abdominal pain, blood passed in the urine or feces or coughed up from the lungs, are always symptoms that should be reported *immediately* to a doctor.

An age of transition

From the age of ten onward the child is growing in physical and mental ability and is becoming increasingly aware of his or her own identity. A common danger at this time is that of overconfidence. The child may feel perfectly able to make a pot of tea or a bacon-and-egg breakfast but the kettle is still heavy and, like the burners, at a difficult height for safe handling. By the same token, the youngster may feel quite able to handle a new bicycle but cannot be expected to appreciate the complexity of the situations that will be encountered on busy urban roads.

In all these situations, the burden of judgement lies with the parents, who should aim for a maximum expression of the child's ability while maintaining a careful – if discreet – level of supervision.

With the new sense of adventure and freedom comes the danger of the challenge – the 'dare' or the game of 'chicken' – to swing higher, spin faster, be last to dash out of the way of the speeding car. Although not easy, the youngster should be encouraged to say, 'No – that's just stupid' rather than feel obliged to follow the crowd.

ALWAYS
- Let the child play hard and encourage him to experiment
- Encourage a responsible attitude to everyday dangers
- Treat all minor injuries without delay
- Seek medical advice if a break or internal injury is suspected

NEVER
- Be over-protective or forget his need for adventure
- Be afraid to seek advice from doctors, teachers or others

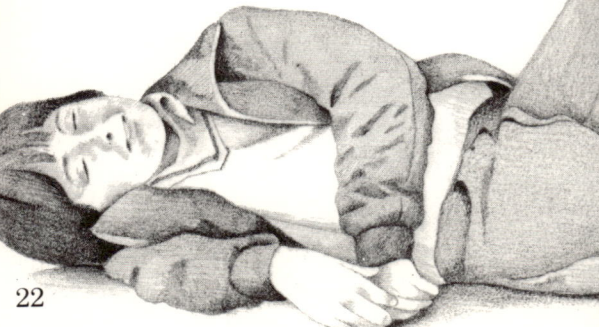

Climbing trees and walls is an expression of the growing child's increasing awareness of his strength and skill. Advise him to be careful but don't inhibit his sense of adventure.

Skateboarding, like cycling, roller-skating and many other activities, has its dangers but these can be minimized by encouraging common sense and insisting on proper protective clothing.

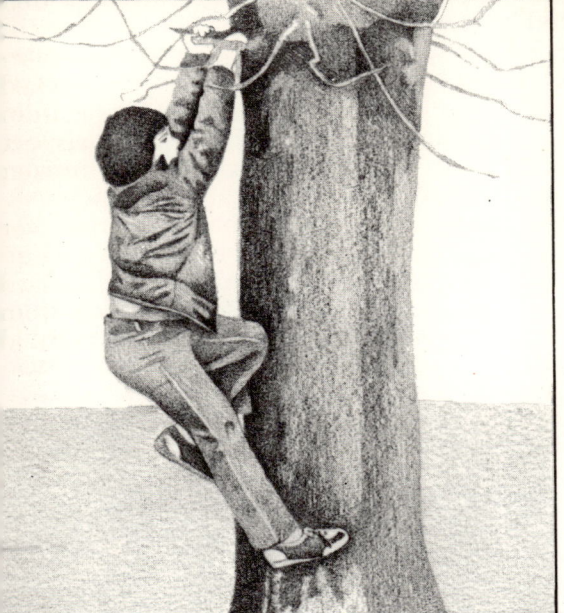
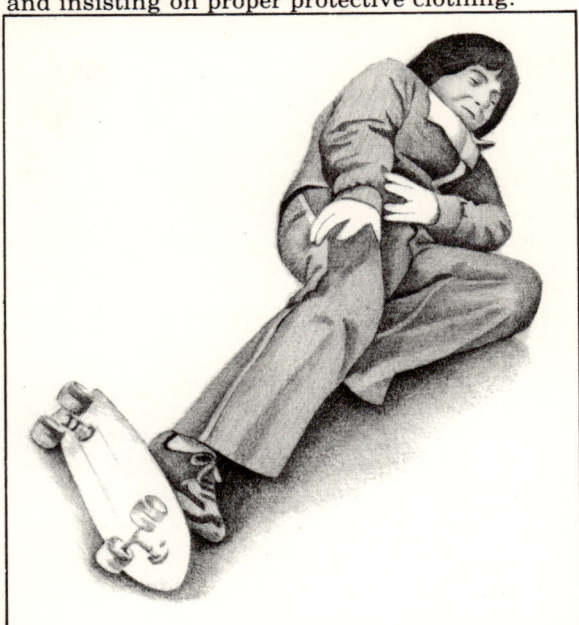

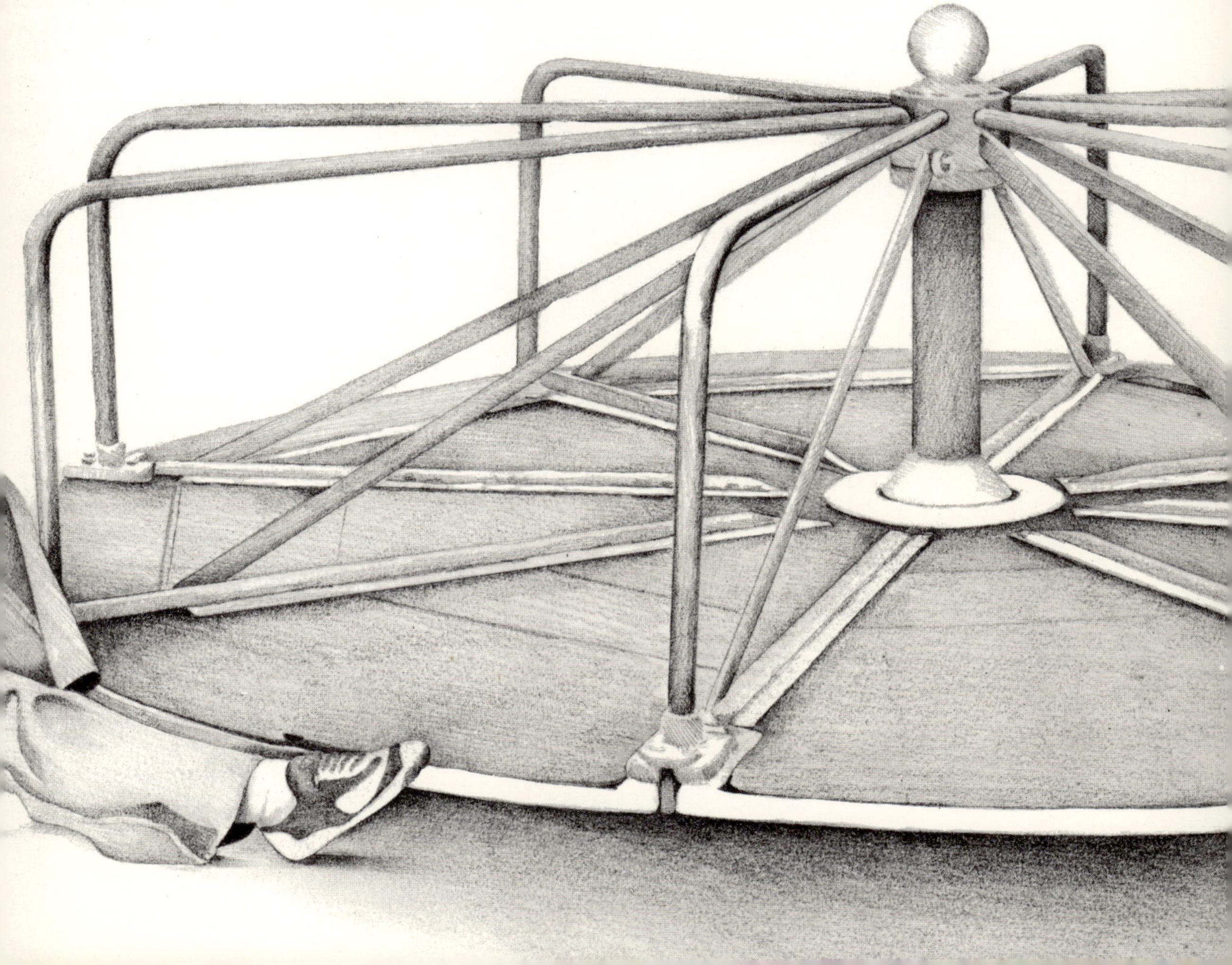

Teenager

By the age of seventeen, the child almost certainly feels that he or she is already an adult and in order to promote this image the young person is likely to undertake any activity that he or she believes to be symbolic of adulthood, largely as a demonstration of maturity. Unfortunately, the skill and judgement which come only from experience are all too often lacking and thus many of these new activities involve potential dangers.

This is particularly true of driving – whether motorcycle or car – and drinking, for teenagers and their friends are coming into increasingly early contact with drink at parties and in restaurants and bars. The games of childhood are also being replaced by more dangerous and adventurous pursuits like rock climbing, skiing and hang-gliding – all of which need expert training and guidance if accidents are to be avoided.

Leading by example

It is difficult, if not impossible, to *tell* teenagers what to do for this is the age of rebellion against authority. But by example and discussion, and by treating their children as adults, parents can still exert an important and lasting influence.

If the parents do not smoke, for example, the children are less likely to adopt the habit. If alcohol has always been used with good sense in the home, a similar mature attitude to drink is far more likely to develop.

Parents can also help minimize risks to their children by insisting on proper driving instruction for the learner and by pointing out the good sense in wearing crash helmets and using seat belts. They can also encourage them to learn to swim well and to learn at least the basics of first aid.

Many, if not most, teenagers are idealistic and parents are more likely to exert positive influence by stressing their responsibilities toward other people than by warning them of the penalties of the law or by trying to impose sanctions at home. The seventeen-year-old *knows* that drinking and driving don't mix, but he is less likely to overindulge if he is made aware of the possibility of killing an innocent victim than if he is simply concerned at being caught by police after an evening drinking.

Other drugs beside alcohol may be tried and while a distinction may be drawn between 'soft' drugs like marijuana, and 'hard' drugs like heroin, *all* are potentially dangerous. The former are not too harmful, though they carry some danger of dependency or desire to experiment further; the latter are all too often killers.

Any excessive use of alcohol or drugs is a form of escapism from the harsher realities of life or even from what some young people feel is a rather pointless existence. Parents should take a continuing, active and genuine interest in their children's lives and should encourage them to express themselves fully both at work and leisure.

However, if a parent does suspect that drug abuse is occurring, the problem must not be ignored. Professional advice should be sought immediately from a doctor or from one of the many advisory organizations.

Above all, remember that the teenage years are the time when young people are discovering their own identity, and they must be allowed the freedom to do so in their own way. Making mistakes is all part of learning, but the majority of young people go through the transition from childhood to adulthood without major problems.

Sensible use of alcohol in the home will equip the young person to deal with social drinking

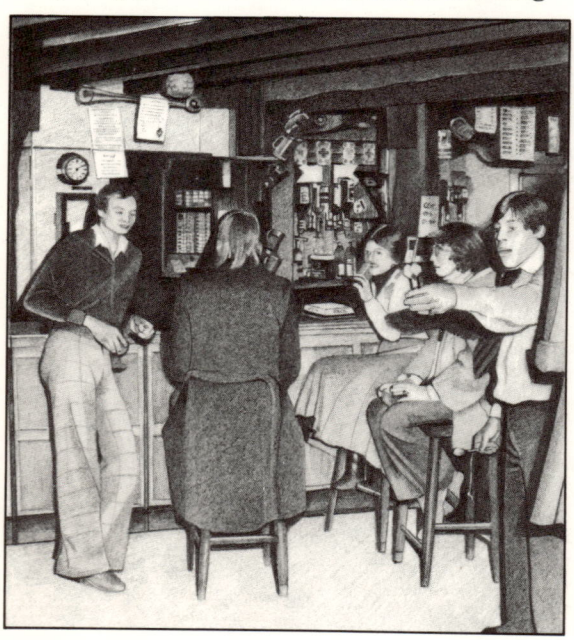

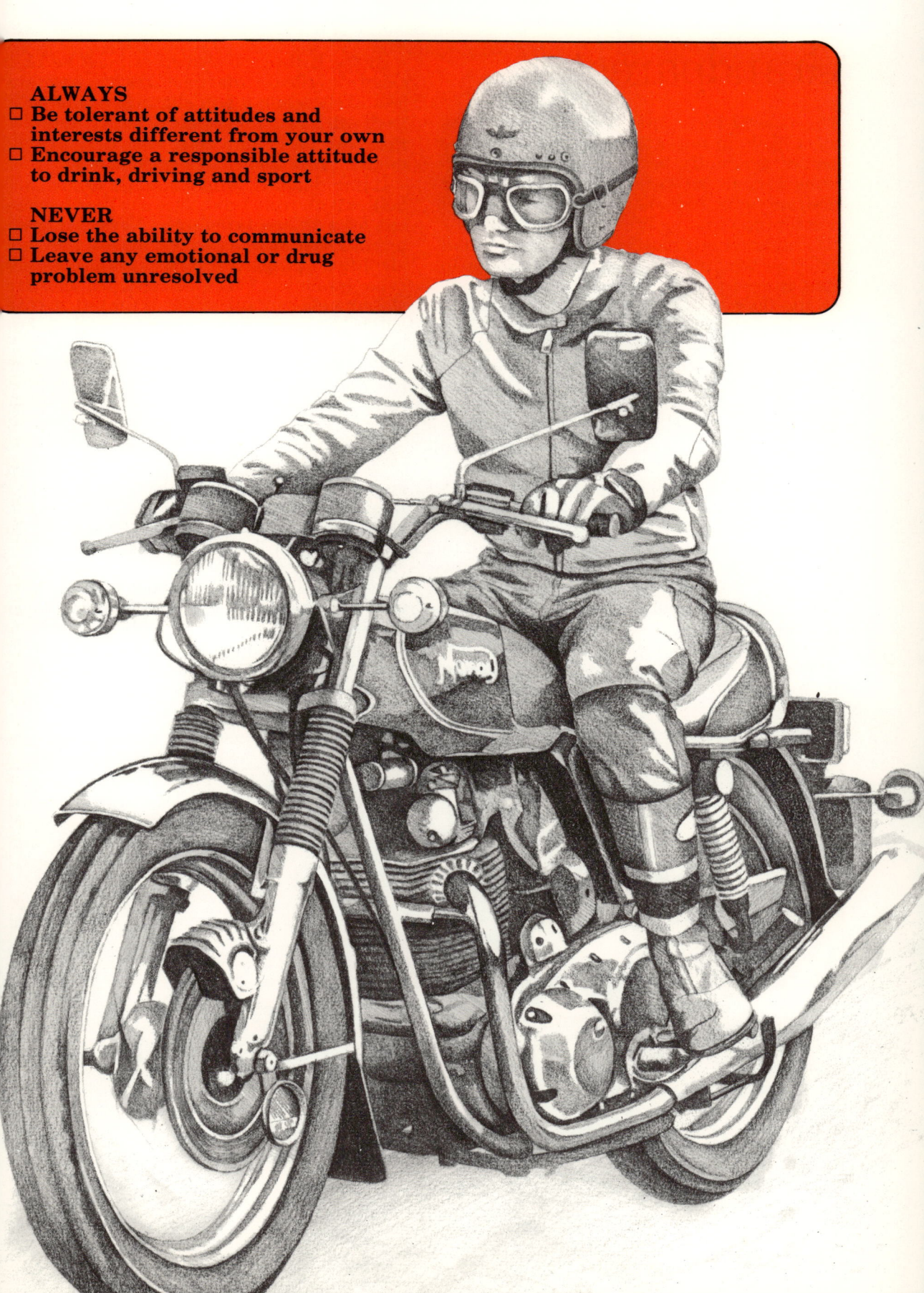

ALWAYS
- Be tolerant of attitudes and interests different from your own
- Encourage a responsible attitude to drink, driving and sport

NEVER
- Lose the ability to communicate
- Leave any emotional or drug problem unresolved

Grandparent

The elderly form one of the three groups most likely to suffer accidents. With age the senses gradually become less acute, reactions become slower, illnesses and bodily malfunctions become more common – all combining to make life more hazardous.

Grandmother almost certainly suffers from defective vision. She thus finds it harder to spot uneven paving stones, steps, loose toys on the floor at home, the edges of mats, the handle of the saucepan. When she does lose her balance, her slower reactions make it more difficult for her to avoid a heavy fall. As she lands, her more brittle bones are more likely to fracture and are then likely to mend more slowly. Added to this, she is quite likely to suffer fits of dizziness which may also cause her to lose her balance.

The same disabilities which put her at such risk of falls also combine to make her more susceptible to burns and scalds. Arthritic hands find it more and more difficult to hold cooking utensils while failing eye-sight increases the risk of spilling hot liquids. Cuts from knives, sharp edges of food tins or broken crockery are all more likely to occur with advancing age and care should be taken to ensure that any minor wounds are treated promptly to avoid complications.

In the bathroom, medicines must be kept clearly labelled so that mistakes in dosage are less likely while a non slip mat in the bath itself will lessen the danger of falls. Handrails near the bath and toilet will help grandmother lower and raise herself safely.

If grandmother cannot manage to open pill bottles with child-proof tops, ask the pharmacist for a different container. Never put them in other containers yourself in case they are identified wrongly at a later date and possibly cause poisoning. Likewise, never let her leave sleeping-pill containers beside the bed, in case she becomes confused and repeatedly takes her normal dosage.

The elderly often have trouble with their feet and many, for instance, find that they can no longer trim their own toenails. If they cannot manage, and you feel unable to help, ask for treatment by a chiropodist.

Outside the home, wet paths, unexpected steps or an ill-lit route to the trashcan are the kind of hazards likely to lead to falls among the elderly. Ask grandmother not to go outside in poor light or in darkness.

As a general comment, it is also worth noting that older people often become quite eccentric about diet, or neglect to make proper meals. This renders them liable to deficiency illnesses which may need to be corrected. By far the best protection is to ensure that the elderly receive regular visits.

Strong medications left on the bedside table are a serious hazard to the absent-minded.

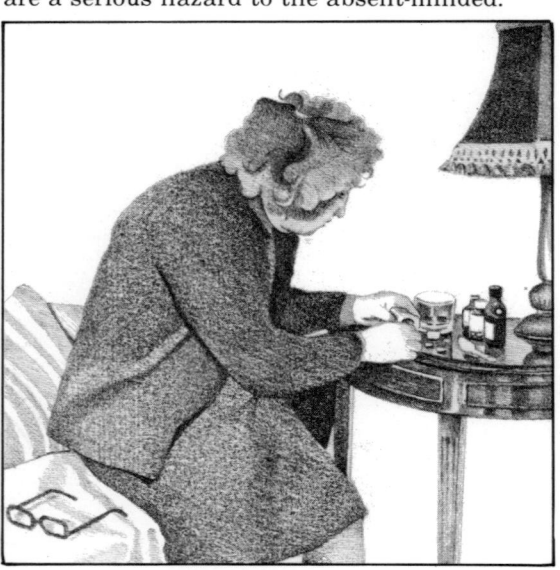

Hypothermia, a dangerous lowering of the body temperature, kills many old people every year.

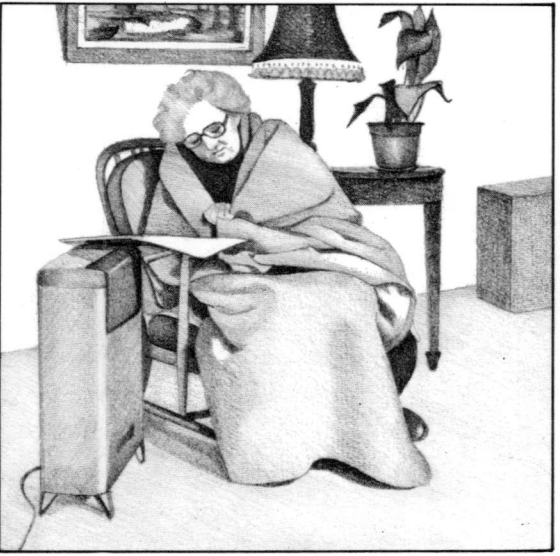

ALWAYS
- ☐ Remember that reactions are slower in elderly people
- ☐ Remember that old bones break easily and mend slowly
- ☐ Guard all open fires
- ☐ Take steps to make household facilities safe for the old

NEVER
- ☐ Put pills into non-standard or wrongly-marked containers
- ☐ Leave sleeping pills beside an elderly person's bed
- ☐ Leave any injury untreated
- ☐ Leave an elderly person alone for long periods

Uncertain balance, imperfect eye-sight and uneven steps are a dangerous combination. Falls while performing household tasks account for a high proportion of accidents suffered by elderly people.

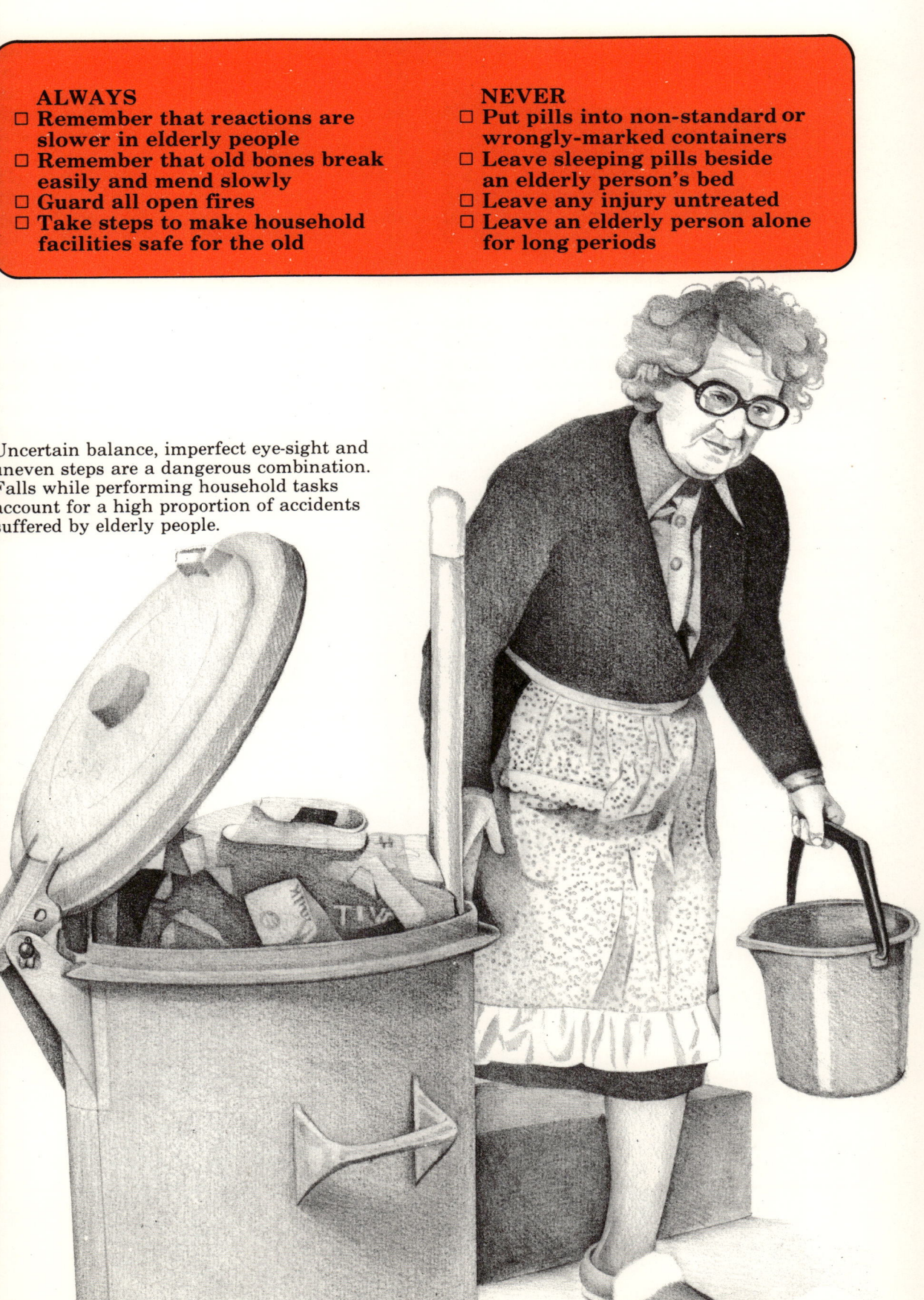

Kitchen

The kitchen is a busy place, particularly when mother is cooking and young children are in the room with her. Electrical and gas appliances are often in use and boiling water and hot fat, sharp implements and poisonous substances are there too. Special care is needed therefore to keep the risk of accidents to a minimum.

On the stove, make sure that all utensils have their handles turned inward where they cannot be accidentally brushed against and tipped over by a passing adult, or pulled over by an inquisitive child. Many stove manufacturers supply guard rails that can be fitted around the edge of the stove so that saucepans cannot be knocked or pulled to the floor.

If you cook by gas, always make absolutely certain that no gas is escaping from an unlit burner. Gas can be a killer, whether it be a build-up of unlit gas suddenly igniting explosively, unlit gas causing suffocation from the carbon monoxide that is present in the town gas in some countries, or just slow suffocation as otherwise non-toxic gas displaces the oxygen we need to breathe.

Most gas used in the home has a distinctive smell, but if there is none then extra care must be taken. Never meddle with gas piping or attempt to install your own.

Many cleaning materials are poisonous and represent a grave hazard to children. Household bleach is an obvious example, but even the disinfectants that are so useful in dilution can be harmful in concentrated form. Keep all such items in cupboards or drawers where small children cannot easily get hold of them.

The same applies to knives and other sharp kitchen implements – and the housewife must take care whenever she is using a knife or when she is handling an opened can with sharp and jagged edges.

Floors should be non-slip but, even when they are, patches of moisture, say from a spilled kettle, can make the surface temporarily slippery. Always mop up spilled liquid immediately.

When the housewife returns from shopping, most of her purchases will be unpacked in the kitchen and the plastic bags which are being used increasingly often are very inviting for a young child to play with. If the bag is put on as a 'hat', the child may quite easily be suffocated – and many are each year. Always keep plastic bags away from children: tear them and dispose of them immediately.

Hot fat can catch fire only too easily. If it does so, *never* try to dowse it with water for that will cause it to spit and spread. Neither should you try to take the blazing pan out of doors. Put a saucepan lid or an asbestos sheet over it to starve the fire of air, or use a domestic fire extinguisher which does not contain water.

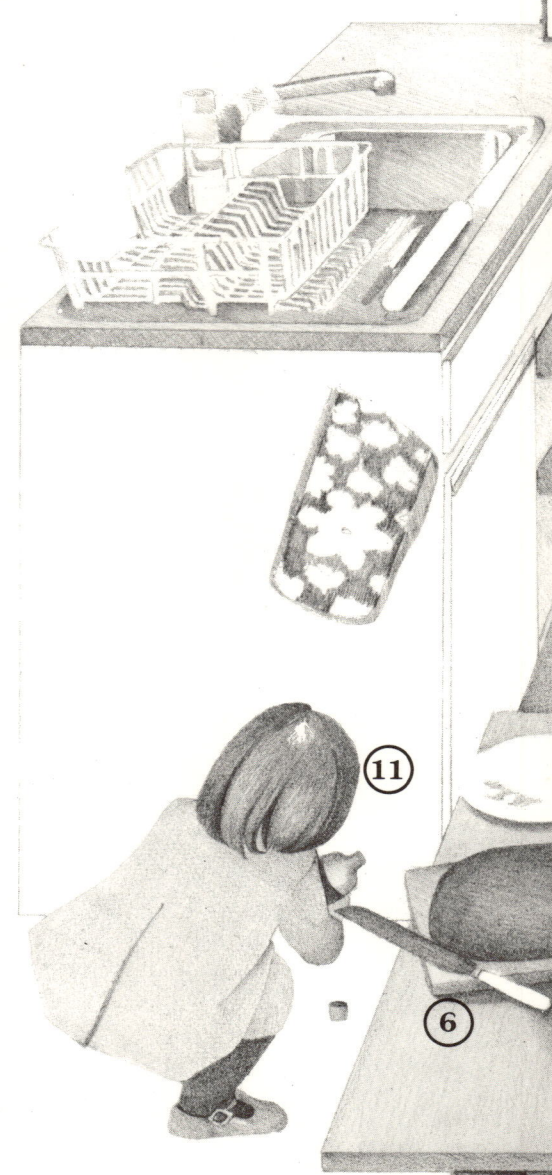

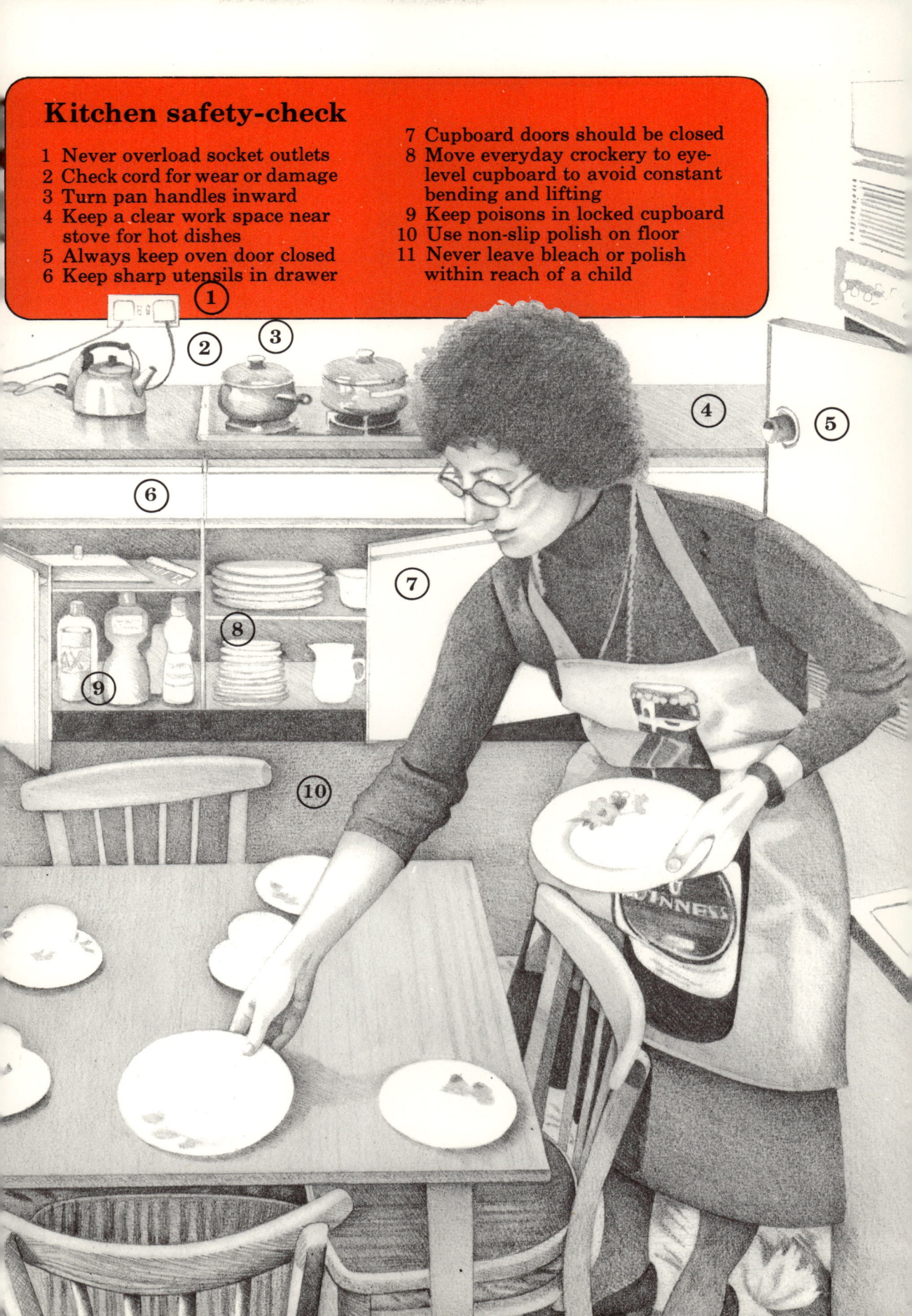

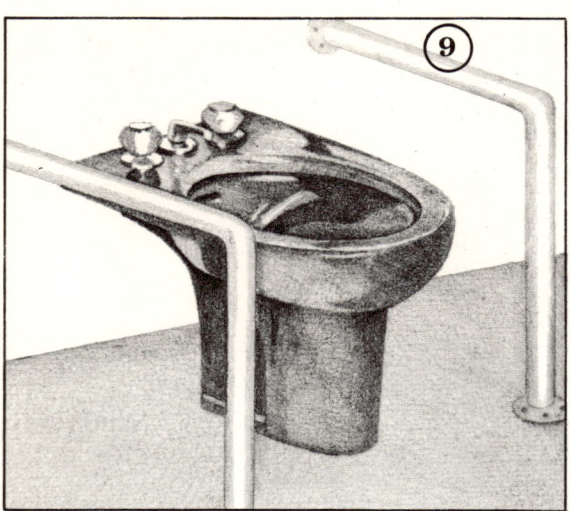

Bathroom safety-check

1. The wall-mounted heater is of approved design but should *not* be over the bath.
2. When running a bath, check the water temperature carefully *before* stepping in.
3. Use a non-slip mat in the bath/shower.
4. Operate an electric shaver only from a properly-installed, insulated socket.
5. Never leave shavers, razors or scissors within reach of a young child.
6. Have a good light over the mirror.
7. Use easily-cleaned, non-slip flooring.
8. Keep all medicines clearly marked and well out of reach of children.
9. Install additional hand-rails to help the elderly and infirm.
10. Attach non-slip backing to all mats.

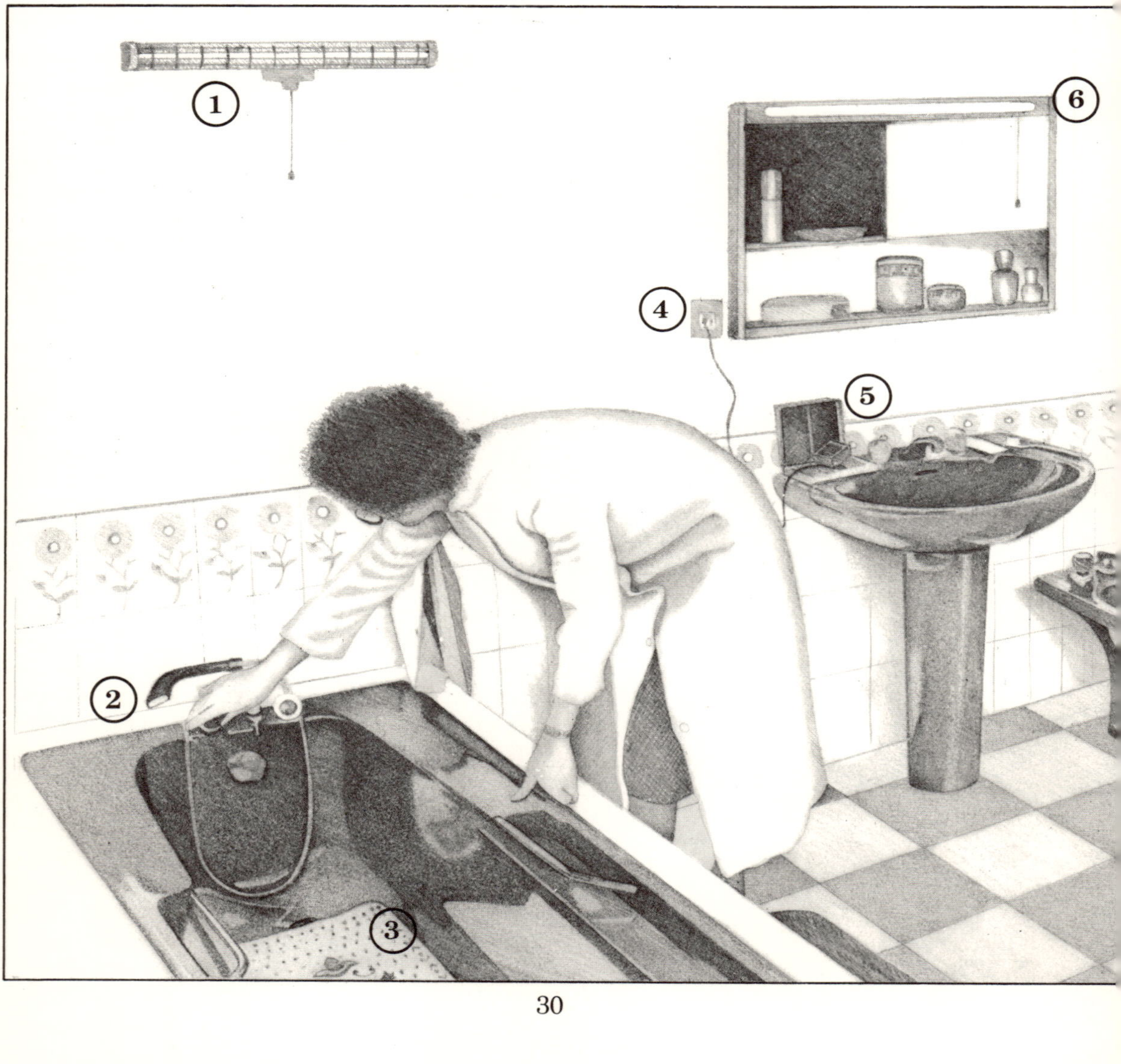

Bathroom

The most common causes of accidents occurring in the bathroom and toilet are falls and electric shock, and yet it is quite remarkable how little effort is made in most households to avoid these most obvious dangers.

Electricity and water form a potentially lethal combination. Water is a very good conductor of electricity so any contact between a person in the bath or shower, and an electrically live object such as a bare wire, faulty switch or the frame of an incompletely grounded heater, *must* be avoided.

If you do have an electric heater in the bathroom, it must be of an approved safe design, be firmly mounted on the wall high enough to be clear of a carelessly flapped towel or piece of clothing, and it must be operated by a pull-cord switch so that a wet hand can never be in danger of touching electrically live parts. Electric shavers, hair dryers and other appliances should be run from individual insulated sockets and not from multiple-outlet adaptor plugs.

Faulty or damaged electric sockets are extremely dangerous in a bathroom and in many countries their presence would represent a direct infringement of statutory building regulations.

Gas water heaters must be maintained in good repair by regular servicing. They must have adequate ventilation, to allow sufficient air to enter for proper combustion, and enough space for the exhaust gases to escape through a flue.

Bathroom mats should have a non-slip backing and, for elderly people whose balance is less certain, a non-slip liner should be provided for the bottom of the bath itself. Firmly fixed grab rails by the bath and lavatory will help to steady the elderly as they rise.

If you have a heated towel rail, make sure that it is positioned well away from any place where bare flesh might accidentally come into contact with it.

The elderly and very young are particularly at risk from burns and scalds, so every precaution must be taken to see that they don't accidentally come into contact with very hot water. For this reason, if you install a shower it is much better to spend a little extra and fit a thermostatically-controlled mixer valve which will ensure that overhot water cannot reach the outlet. When running a bath or shower, it is wiser to run the cold tap first.

Medicines are often kept in the bathroom and it is essential that they are stored where they cannot be reached by children who might mistake them for candy. The best place is in a locked cabinet high enough on the wall to be out of a child's reach. Never keep medicines from which the label is missing, and do not keep any pills left over after an illness is cured. Clear labelling is especially important for elderly people whose eyesight may be failing and who can easily take the wrong medication – or too large a dose of the right one.

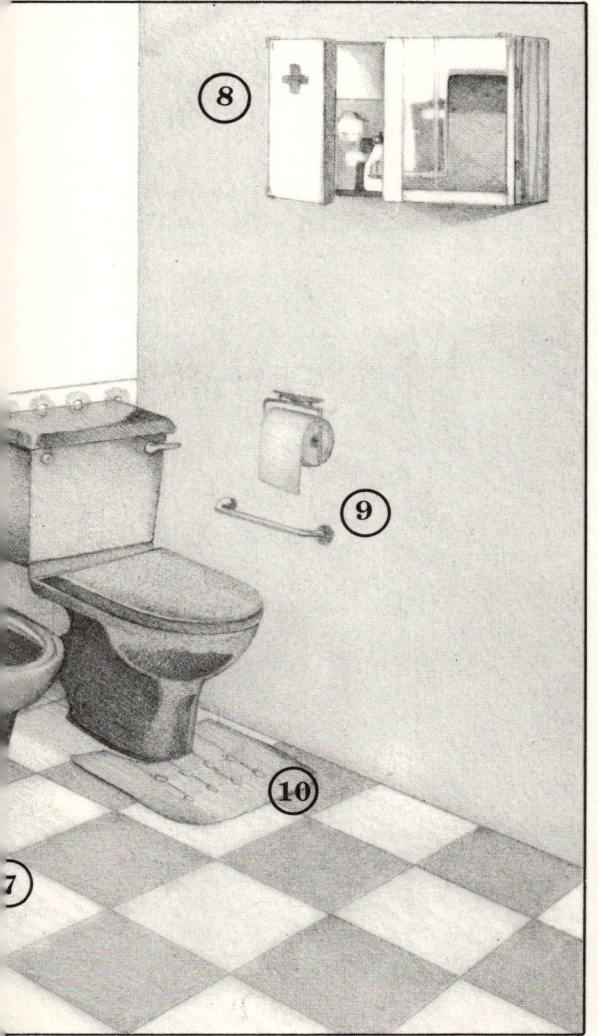

Stairs

Stairs are an obvious hazard in any house, for people of any age but particularly for the very old and the very young. Stair carpets *must* be securely fixed so that they cannot slip. Any holes or worn patches must either be covered safely or the whole carpet should be shifted up or down to move the worn piece to a vertical riser between steps so that feet cannot catch and cause a fall. Always keep the stairs clear of any loose objects such as toys, for they can easily turn into 'roller skates' for the unsuspecting.

Stair rails must be firmly fixed – on both sides if possible so that elderly people can steady themselves with both hands. Open bannisters allow more light on to the stairs than do closed ones but the bannisters should not be so widely spaced that a child could climb through and fall into the stairwell. In any case, stairs must be well-lit, as must steps between adjoining rooms.

Additional protection can be gained by having a low-wattage electric light burning on the landing throughout the night. The cost is very small and the light ensures that nobody moving around in the night half-asleep will trip over furniture or, worse still, down the stairs.

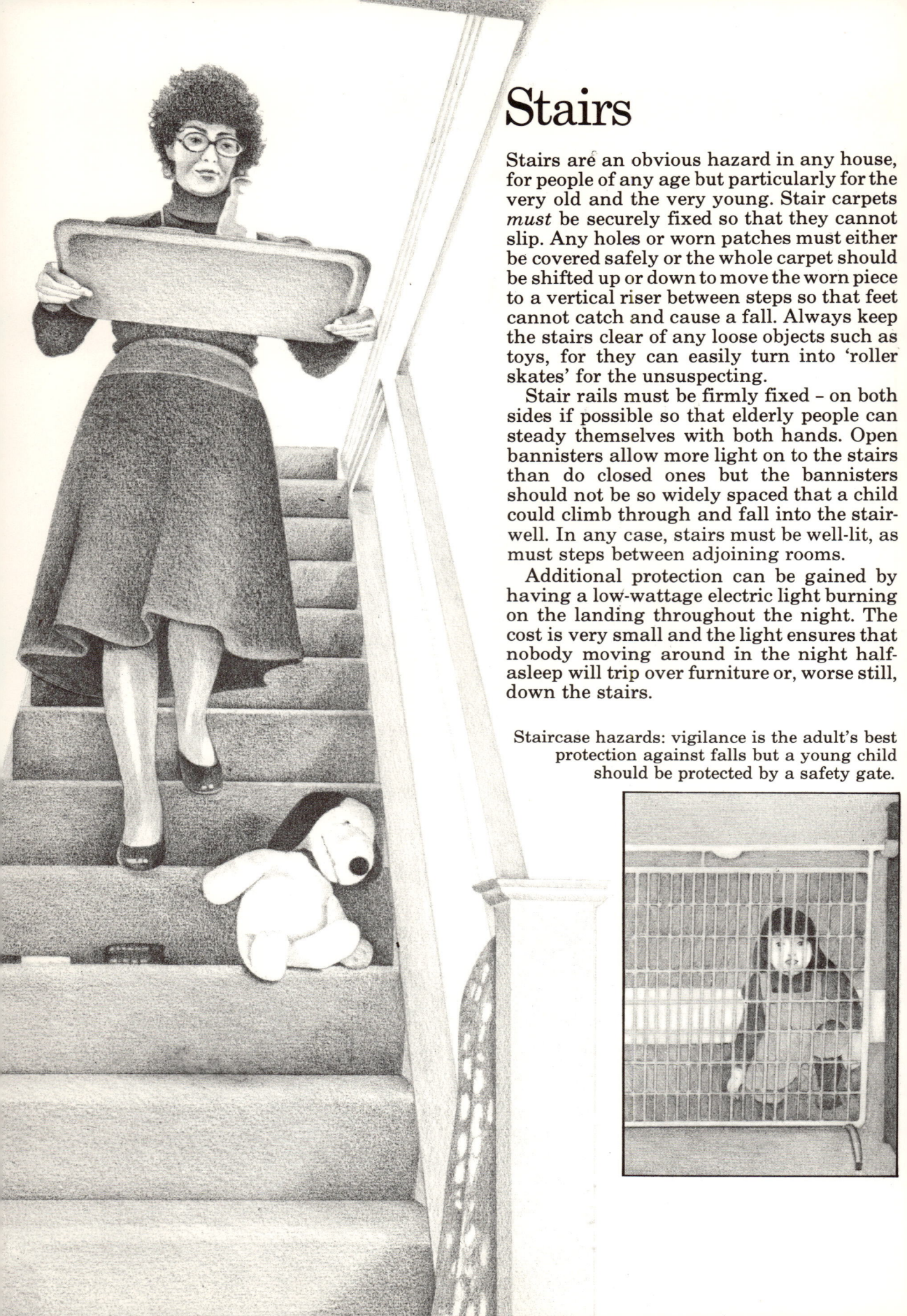

Staircase hazards: vigilance is the adult's best protection against falls but a young child should be protected by a safety gate.

Bedroom

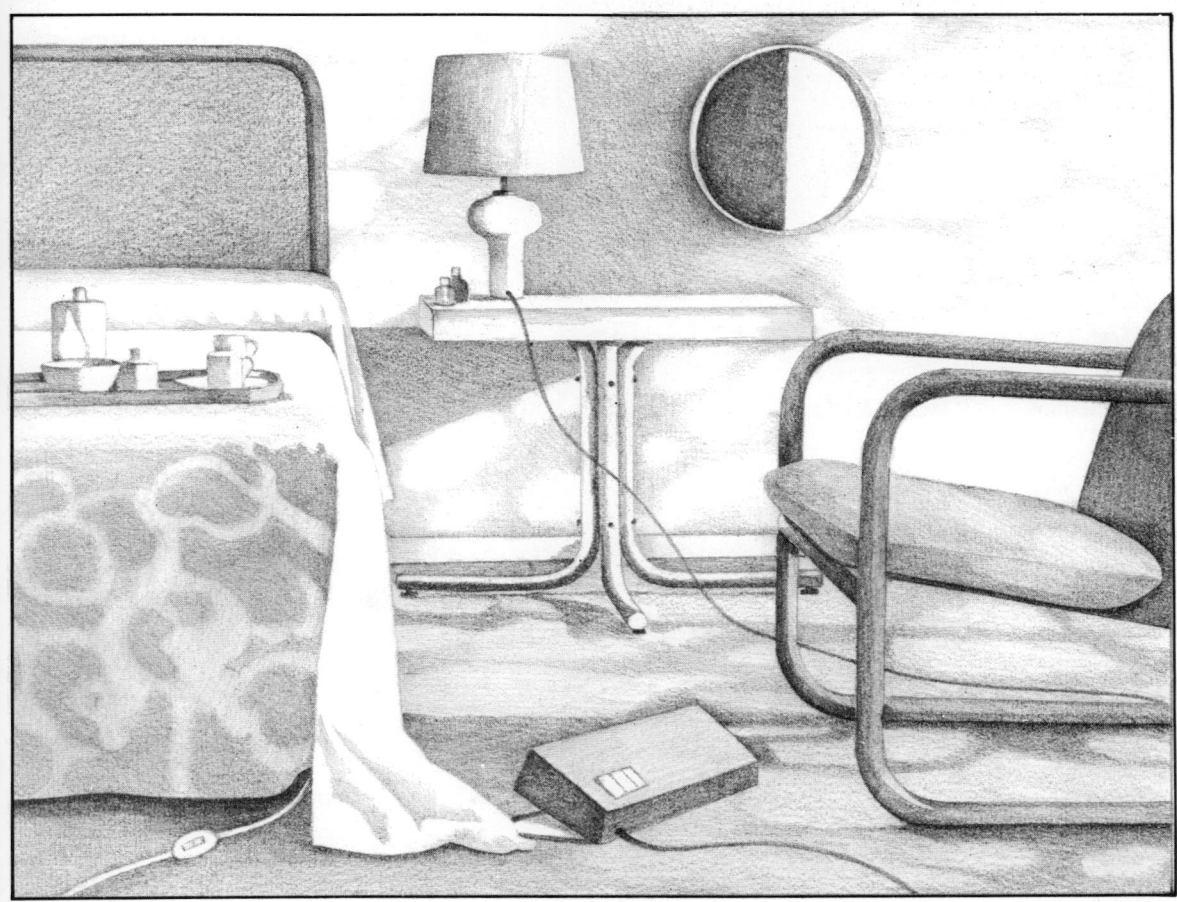

In the bedroom, electrical appliances must be used with the greatest care. Electric blankets, for instance, must be regularly and professionally serviced in accordance with the maker's instructions and they should never be used by anybody, very young or very old, who is likely to wet the bed and short-circuit the blanket. Also, remember not to leave an underblanket switched on after you get into bed unless the instructions expressly say that this is permissible.

An enclosed fan heater is preferable to an open electric heater, gas heater or – most dangerous of all – a kerosene heater, because there is no risk of clothing or bedding touching anything which might set it alight. If you use a heater of any kind, do not place it close to curtains or hanging clothes and do not hang clothes above it to air.

Windows represent one of the main dangers in a child's bedroom – particularly where a bed or table enables the youngster to climb close to the glass. The window should be provided with a safety catch so that the child cannot open it far enough to fall out. Several types of catch are readily available although a simple wood block fixed to the frame will serve just as well in the case of a sash window. Safety bars across the full width of the window afford an added measure of protection – particularly if the window is in such a position that a child could fall against it.

One of the most serious domestic hazards facing young children is the risk of poisoning by medicines left carelessly about in the parents' bedroom. Many modern drugs, and particularly sleeping pills and tranquilizers, are brightly colored: to a child they look exactly like candy – sometimes fatally so.

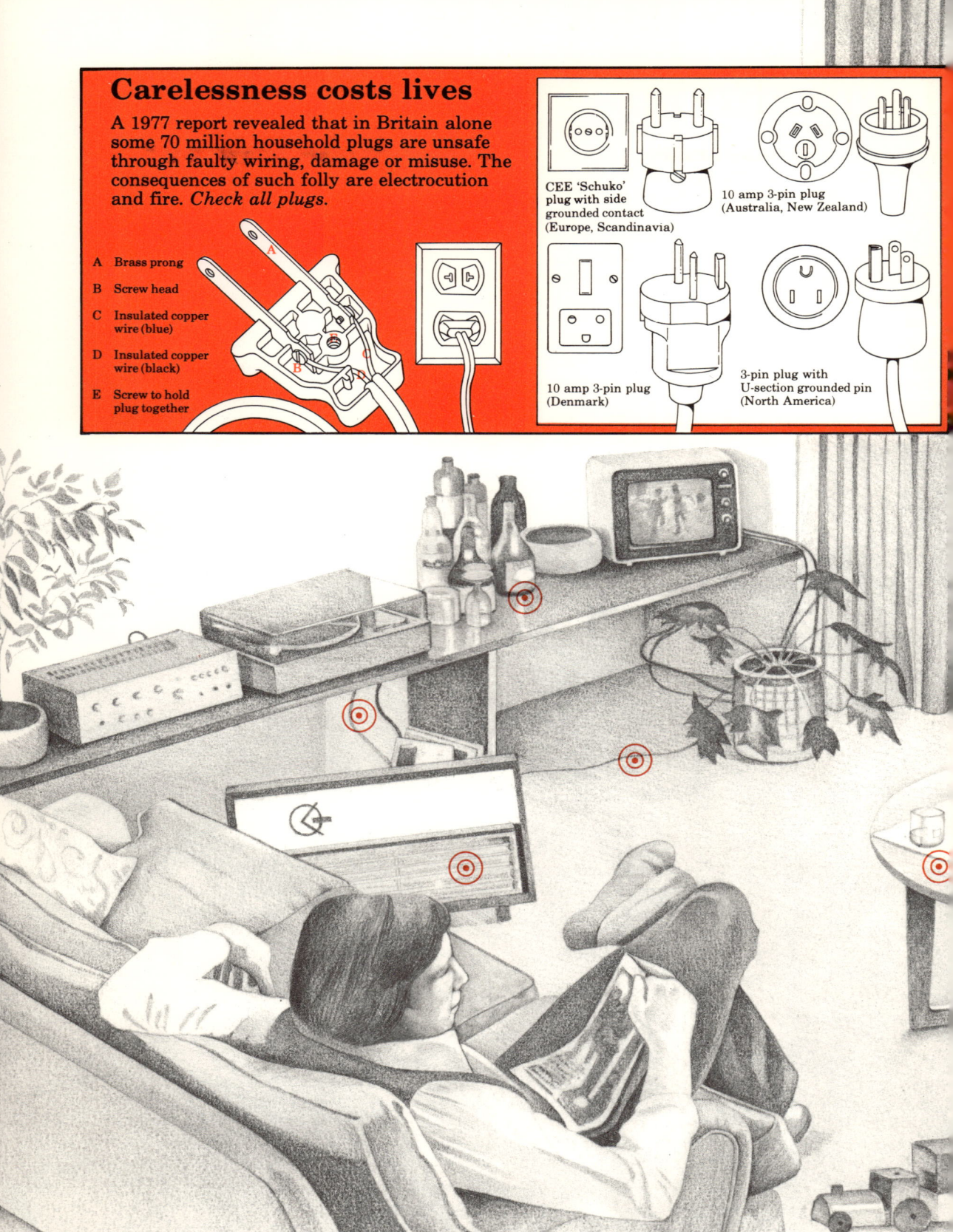

Carelessness costs lives

A 1977 report revealed that in Britain alone some 70 million household plugs are unsafe through faulty wiring, damage or misuse. The consequences of such folly are electrocution and fire. *Check all plugs.*

A   Brass prong
B   Screw head
C   Insulated copper wire (blue)
D   Insulated copper wire (black)
E   Screw to hold plug together

CEE 'Schuko' plug with side grounded contact (Europe, Scandinavia)

10 amp 3-pin plug (Australia, New Zealand)

10 amp 3-pin plug (Denmark)

3-pin plug with U-section grounded pin (North America)

Living Room

Much of one's time for relaxation is spent in the living room, and it is therefore often the warmest and most comfortably furnished room in the house. Yet here too lie dangers.

Many living rooms have polished linoleum or wooden floors. In themselves, these can be dangerous, but they are even more likely to cause falls if mats or rugs are placed over them. If you must put a rug on a polished floor, attach it to a non-slip backing material. Carpets covering a large floor area are not likely to slip, but they can develop worn patches over which the unwary may trip. Repair the worn parts or turn the carpet round so that the worn area is either covered by furniture or is in the least frequented part of the room.

A wide variety of electrical appliances, including television sets, record players, lamps and heaters, are to be found in the living room and it is important to have enough properly wired and grounded wall sockets, preferably one for each item, and to avoid trailing wires. Never take the back off a television set, even if unplugged – a high voltage charge may remain.

◉ Living room danger points

The fireplace is the focal point of many living rooms, so ensure that the fire is adequately guarded. An open coal fire, a gas fire or an open electric heater should be protected by a fine-mesh fireguard that can be securely fixed to the wall.

As a further precaution, do not place a mirror or a small clock above the fireplace, or people will be encouraged to stand unnecessarily close to the fire. If you are airing clothes, never leave them on the fireguard where they may catch fire, or put them where a child might push the clothes-horse into the source of the heat.

If you have one living area combining sitting and dining space, be sure that knives and other sharp implements are kept in a drawer where children are not tempted to grab them. Similarly, if you have alcoholic drink in the dining area, keep it safely out of reach of children – preferably in a locked cupboard. An excessive intake of alcohol will make an adult ill; in a young child it can cause death.

With small children around, it is wise too to see that drinking glasses are kept in a cupboard, safe from breakage and the consequent risk of serious cuts. In general, it is wise to keep *all* ornaments out of reach.

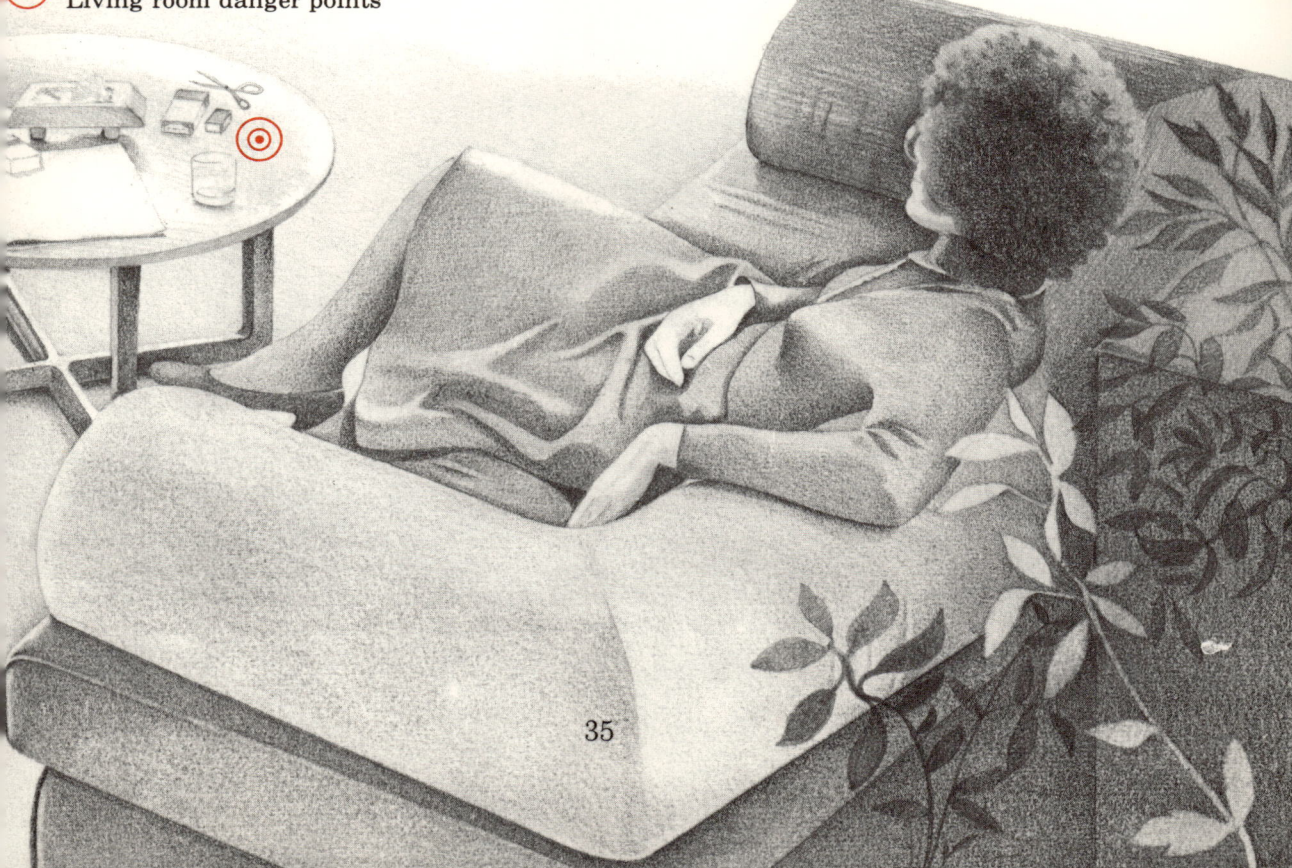

Garage and Workshop

More people than ever before are 'do-it-yourself' enthusiasts, tackling jobs around the home for which in the past they would have called in an expert – the carpenter or plumber, glazier or electrician. And never before have so many tools and gadgets, chemicals, plastics, resins and solvents been readily available to make the task of doing-it-yourself easier.

This revolution, however, means that the place where these tools and materials are most often used and stored – the garage or workshop – is a distinct danger zone where accidents are concerned. The most obvious dangers come from sharp tools: chisels, saws, screwdrivers, gouges and the like. The cuts and puncture wounds caused by their careless use form a high proportion of home accidents requiring hospital treatment.

Safe Workshop Practice

The risks can be minimized by following a few simple rules. Always, for instance, work in a good light: the work bench, particularly, should be well-lit. Use tools with both hands behind the cutting edge, work away from the body, and always carry them point downwards. Put them away immediately after use: it is all too easy, for children especially, to suffer cuts from sharp tools left lying around. Keep children out of the way when working: *in more than one third of do-it-yourself accidents it is the child watching, rather than the adult, who is hurt.* Electrical tools and their cords should always be kept in good repair and cracked plugs and worn wires replaced immediately. If an extension cord is used, insure that the joint has its socket towards the power source and the plug towards the appliance. Read the maker's instructions carefully before using any new power tool. Protect the eyes when doing jobs where sparks or splinters may fly. Switch off and unplug before you start mending or adjusting electrical equipment.

The chemical hazard

Many of the chemicals now used in the garden, workshop and garage need most careful use, storage and disposal. They should be kept in their original containers, *clearly labelled* and firmly closed and they should be stored in a safe place out of the reach of children. The manufacturers' instructions should be carefully followed, especially those about smoking, avoiding contact with the eyes and skin, or washing your hands before eating. Failure to do so can result in explosion, fire or poisoning.

Other potentially dangerous chemicals are also likely to be stored in the garage or workshop, notably garden chemical fertilizers, insecticides and weedkillers. These, too, should be kept in their original containers: *never*, for example, put weedkiller in a soft-drink bottle or food container, and keep well away from children.

The garage or workshop needs to be well-ventilated so that poisonous fumes and inflammable vapors can disperse quickly. The car engine should never be kept running in the garage: the exhaust emits poisonous carbon monoxide which can be fatal. Take great care too in handling anti-freeze mixtures, brake fluid and gasoline. For tasks carried out about the garage and workshop, follow this straight-forward procedure: think out carefully what you are going to do, get out all the tools and materials you will need before you start and while you are at work, concentrate on what you are doing, especially when using knives, chisels and saws.

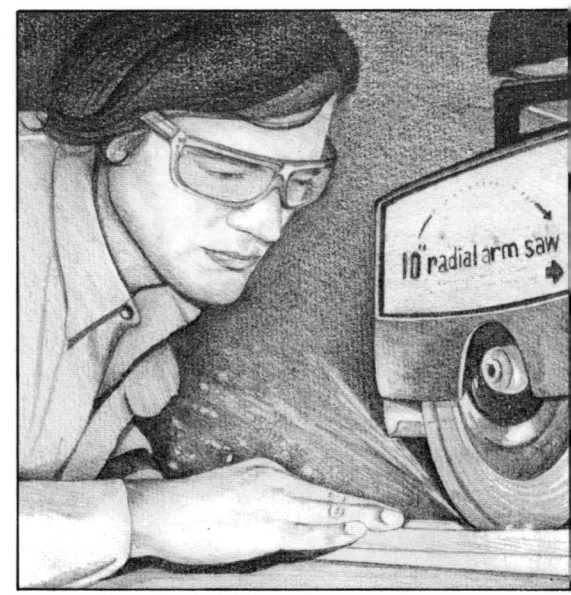

ALWAYS
- Wear safety goggles when using sanders, saws or wire brushes
- Wear a face mask when spraying paint, varnish or chemicals
- Read and observe makers' warnings on tools and chemical products
- Work in good light
- Keep tools sharp and in good repair

NEVER
- Place dangerous chemicals in 'innocent' looking containers
- Leave sharp tools within the reach of a child
- Use vaporizing chemicals in confined spaces

When using power tools, always wear goggles or safety glasses to protect the eyes from flying particles. Nasal passages, throat and lungs should be protected from paint and other finely sprayed fluids by use of a filter mask.

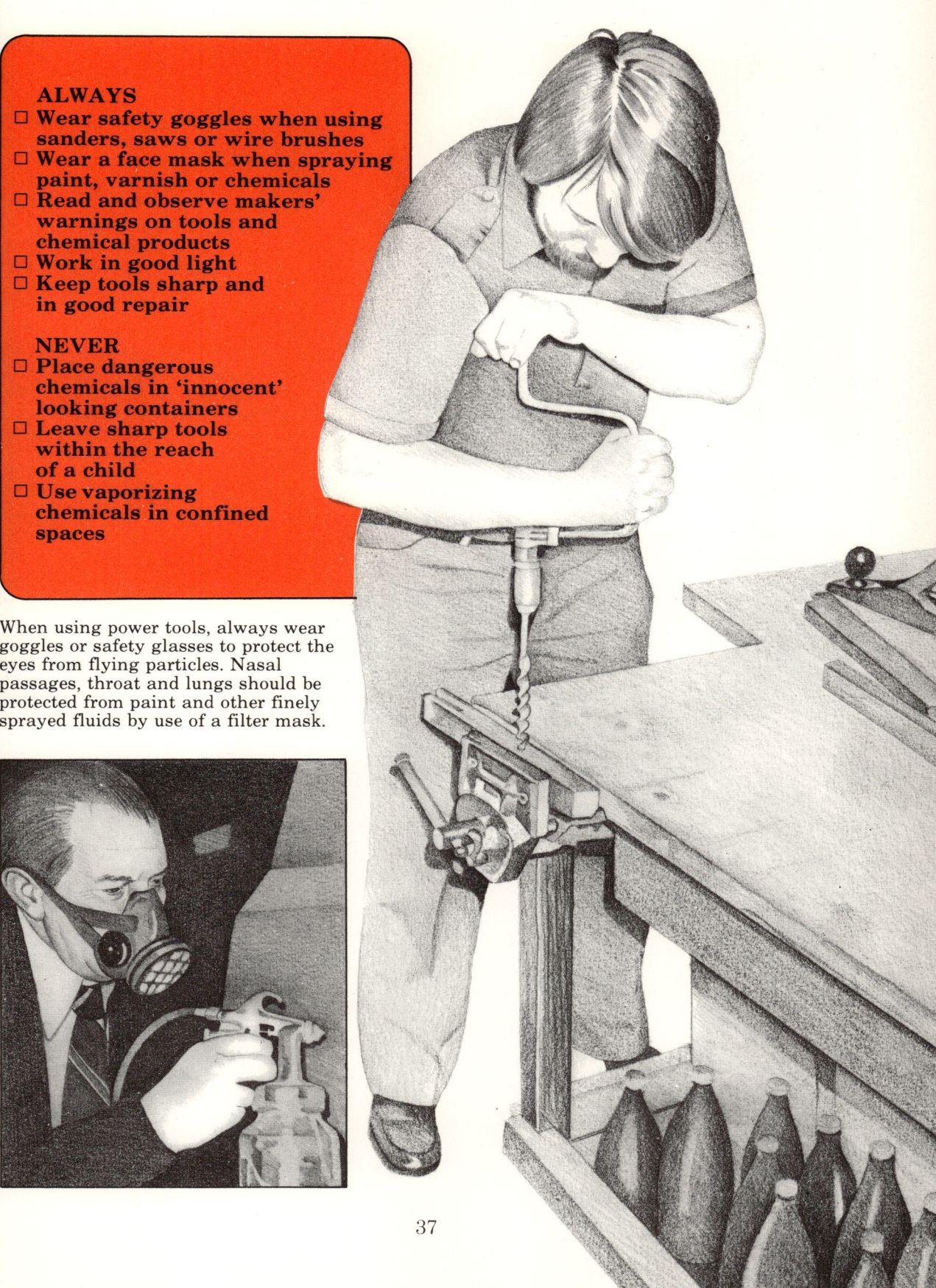

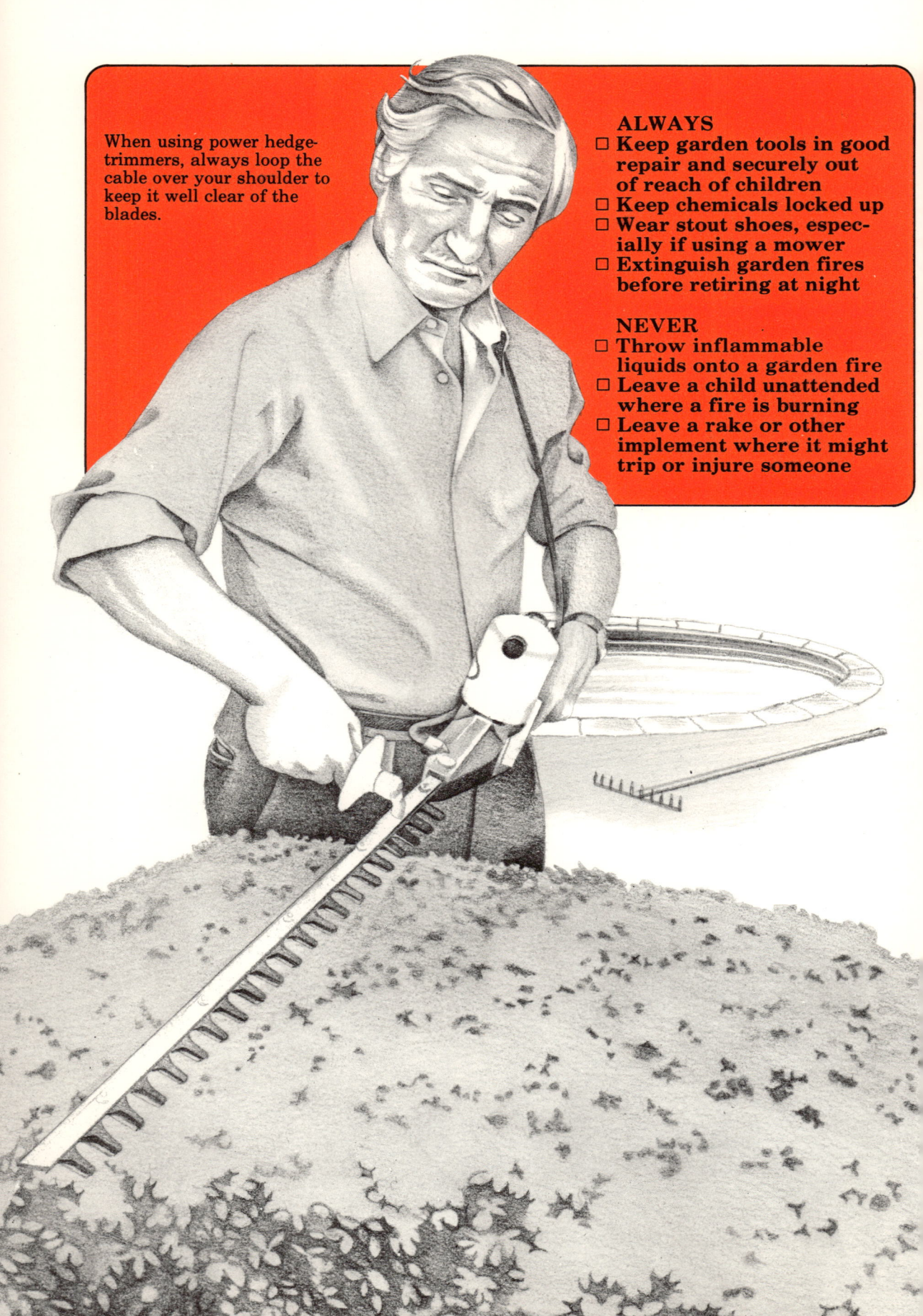

When using power hedge-trimmers, always loop the cable over your shoulder to keep it well clear of the blades.

ALWAYS
- Keep garden tools in good repair and securely out of reach of children
- Keep chemicals locked up
- Wear stout shoes, especially if using a mower
- Extinguish garden fires before retiring at night

NEVER
- Throw inflammable liquids onto a garden fire
- Leave a child unattended where a fire is burning
- Leave a rake or other implement where it might trip or injure someone

Garden

A large proportion of home accidents each year happen in the garden so, when you finally get down to doing those simple jobs you've been meaning to do for weeks, one thing to remember right at the start is not to over-exert yourself in a sudden rush of reckless enthusiasm. Unless you are used to physical activity, there is a risk of back strain, torn muscles or even, possibly, heart attack.

When burning leaves, cuttings or other garden rubbish, you should always use a properly built incinerator. A small amount of kerosene may be used in order to start the fire but always replace the cap on the can, and remove it to a safe distance, *before* lighting the fire. *Never* throw inflammable liquids onto a burning fire. Keep children and pets at a safe distance at all times and make sure that the fire is properly extinguished before you finally go indoors.

If you have an electric lawn-mower, it should always be handled with great care. Never use it when it's raining or when the grass is wet, and don't leave it out in the rain. The cable should be a bright color, easy to see, so that there is less likelihood of running the mower over it. Check all cables and fitments carefully before you use the machine. Never cut the grass by pulling an electric mower towards you, and don't pick it up while it is running.

Rotary mowers have an added danger: on wet grass, and particularly on a sloping lawn, they are difficult to control. Never stand downhill of the mower and always wear stout shoes or boots. Clear away any sticks or stones from the lawn before you start, because with the tips of the rotor blades moving at 200 miles an hour anything coming into contact with them can be flung far and hard. Always stop the motor before leaving a mower unattended and before pushing it along paths.

Electric hedge trimmers should always be used with the cable trailing over the opposite shoulder to the hand they are held in to avoid any risk of cutting through the cable.

Don't leave garden shears lying about on the path to be trodden on. That goes for all your other garden tools as well – treading on the garden rake is no laughing matter.

Knives and shears should always be stored with their blades in the closed position.

Check fences to make sure that there are no protruding nails or splinters. If you have an ornamental garden pond, remember that a toddler can drown in only three inches of water, so don't underestimate the danger. Children should be supervised at all times in the garden. Check garden swing fittings which may have corroded or rotted during the winter months. Deckchairs too after winter storage should be checked over. Show children the right way to open and close them to avoid trapped fingers.

When staking plants, make sure the stakes are at least four feet high and easy to see. If you bend down to examine a plant without seeing a stake, you could suffer an unpleasant face or eye injury. If in doubt, attach pieces of paper or cloth to the tops of the canes to make them more conspicuous.

Power mowers are a boon if large areas are to be cut but always wear stout shoes to protect the toes, and clear away all loose stones.

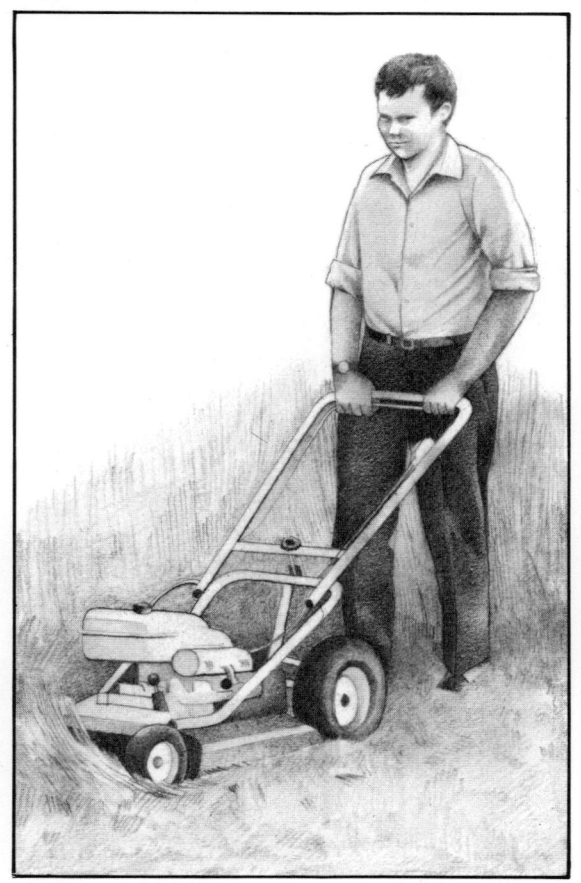

Toxic Plants

Even the most innocent-looking garden may contain a surprising number of flowers and shrubs which are poisonous to some degree. Many cause only mild symptoms if eaten but some are extremely dangerous and children must be taught *never* to eat the leaves, flowers or berries of any plant, no matter how enticing it may look.

Many a garden is brightened in summer by the golden flowers of the laburnum tree – but it is as deadly as it is beautiful and the seed pods contain tiny kidney-shaped beans that are very tempting to a child. Other common, and poisonous, trees and shrubs include yew, holly, mistletoe, wisteria and almost all varieties of laurel. Aconite, or monkshood, is a very poisonous garden plant and lupins, azaleas, delphiniums, lily-of-the-valley and many others are potentially dangerous. Even food plants may have some dangerous parts: rhubarb leaves, tomato leaves and stems and potato leaves and stems all contain toxic substances.

A number of common indoor plants should also be treated with care. Poinsettia, often kept as a houseplant, has a resinous sap which can cause a blistering rash unless washed off the skin immediately. Other indoor hazards include the 'Jerusalem Cherry,' 'Dumb Cane,' and oleanders.

Out in the woods and fields, all plants should be regarded as potentially dangerous. Mushrooms and toadstools account for many cases of poisoning every year so leave well alone unless you know the safe from the unsafe species. Of the common wild flowers, the nightshades, foxgloves, hemlock, meadow saffron and Jack-in-the-Pulpit, are all poisonous while the sap from crowfoots and clematis can cause dermatitis. A more serious skin reaction is caused by poison ivy. Like poison sumac and poison oak, it has a poisonous sap running through the entire plant. If burned, its fumes can produce irritation to the eyes and respiratory tract. The poison can be spread by clothing and even by petting animals that have been in contact with the leaves.

If poisoning of a child, or adult, is suspected, take the casualty to a hospital as quickly as possible – taking along also a sample of whatever plant has been eaten.

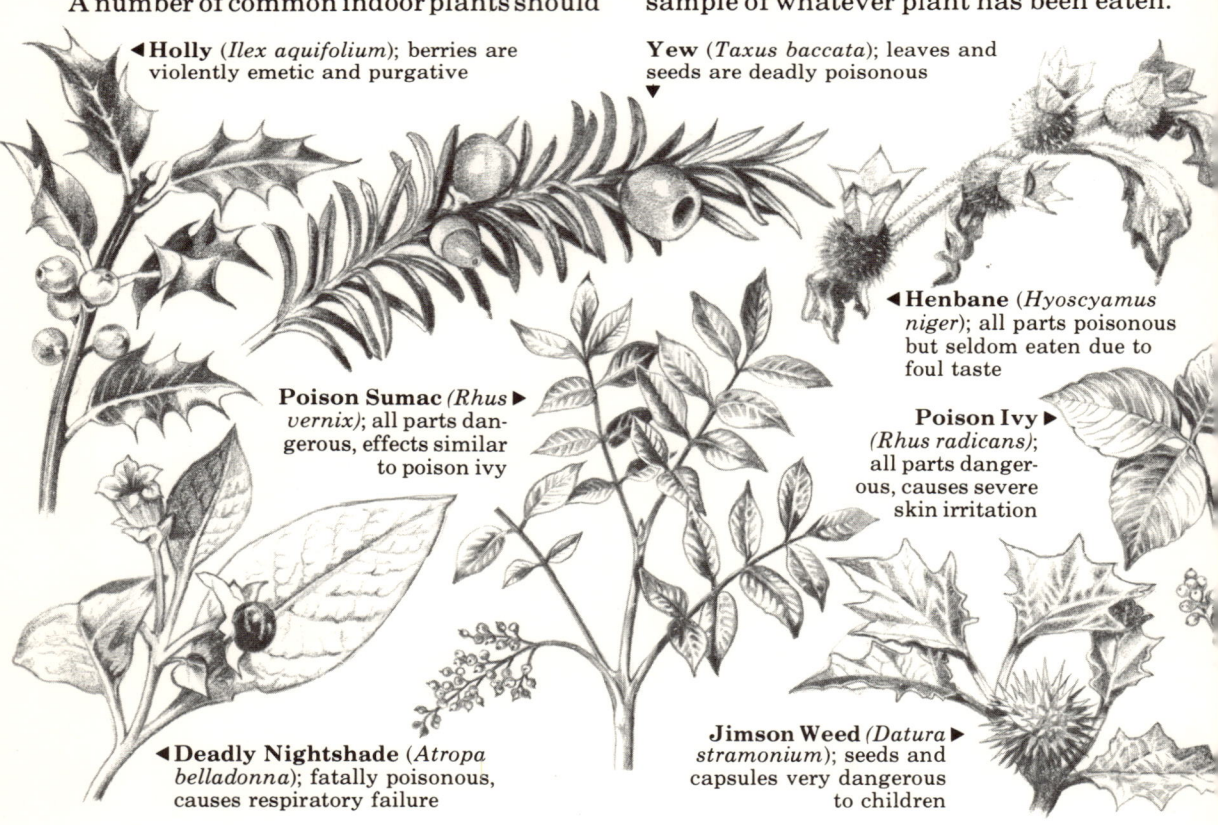

◀ **Holly** (*Ilex aquifolium*); berries are violently emetic and purgative

Yew (*Taxus baccata*); leaves and seeds are deadly poisonous

◀ **Henbane** (*Hyoscyamus niger*); all parts poisonous but seldom eaten due to foul taste

Poison Sumac (*Rhus vernix*) ▶; all parts dangerous, effects similar to poison ivy

Poison Ivy ▶ (*Rhus radicans*); all parts dangerous, causes severe skin irritation

◀ **Deadly Nightshade** (*Atropa belladonna*); fatally poisonous, causes respiratory failure

Jimson Weed (*Datura* ▶ *stramonium*); seeds and capsules very dangerous to children

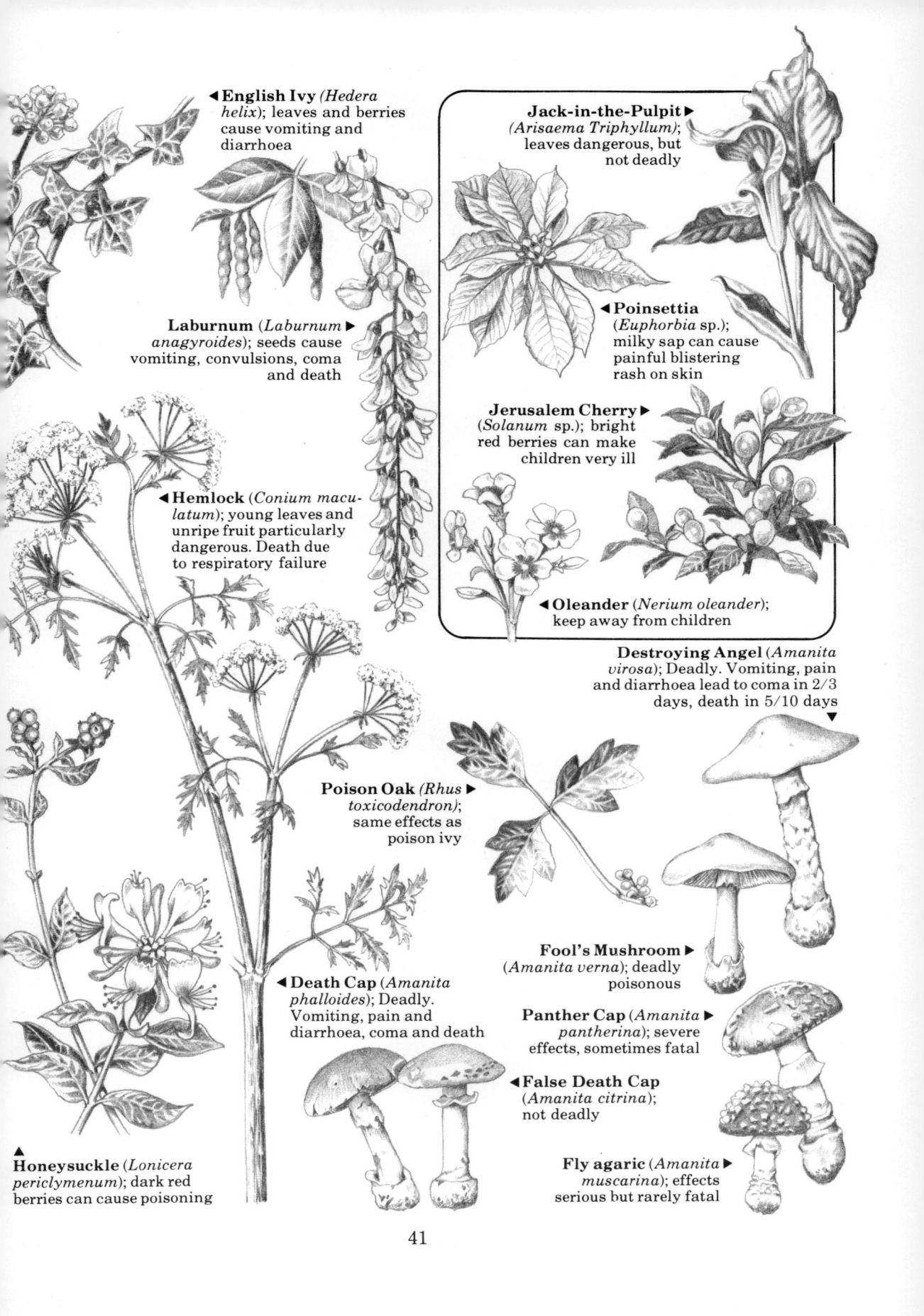

◀ **English Ivy** (*Hedera helix*); leaves and berries cause vomiting and diarrhoea

Jack-in-the-Pulpit ▶ (*Arisaema Triphyllum*); leaves dangerous, but not deadly

Laburnum (*Laburnum* ▶ *anagyroides*); seeds cause vomiting, convulsions, coma and death

◀ **Poinsettia** (*Euphorbia* sp.); milky sap can cause painful blistering rash on skin

Jerusalem Cherry ▶ (*Solanum* sp.); bright red berries can make children very ill

◀ **Hemlock** (*Conium maculatum*); young leaves and unripe fruit particularly dangerous. Death due to respiratory failure

◀ **Oleander** (*Nerium oleander*); keep away from children

Destroying Angel (*Amanita virosa*); Deadly. Vomiting, pain and diarrhoea lead to coma in 2/3 days, death in 5/10 days

Poison Oak (*Rhus* ▶ *toxicodendron*); same effects as poison ivy

Fool's Mushroom ▶ (*Amanita verna*); deadly poisonous

◀ **Death Cap** (*Amanita phalloides*); Deadly. Vomiting, pain and diarrhoea, coma and death

Panther Cap (*Amanita* ▶ *pantherina*); severe effects, sometimes fatal

◀ **False Death Cap** (*Amanita citrina*); not deadly

Fly agaric (*Amanita* ▶ *muscarina*); effects serious but rarely fatal

▲ **Honeysuckle** (*Lonicera periclymenum*); dark red berries can cause poisoning

The First Aid Kit

STERILE GAUZE, COTTON, ANTISEPTIC SOLUTION and PRE-PACKED ANTISEPTIC WIPES are basic requirements for cleaning minor wounds prior to bandaging ANTISEPTIC CREAM soothes cuts and grazes stings and rashes.

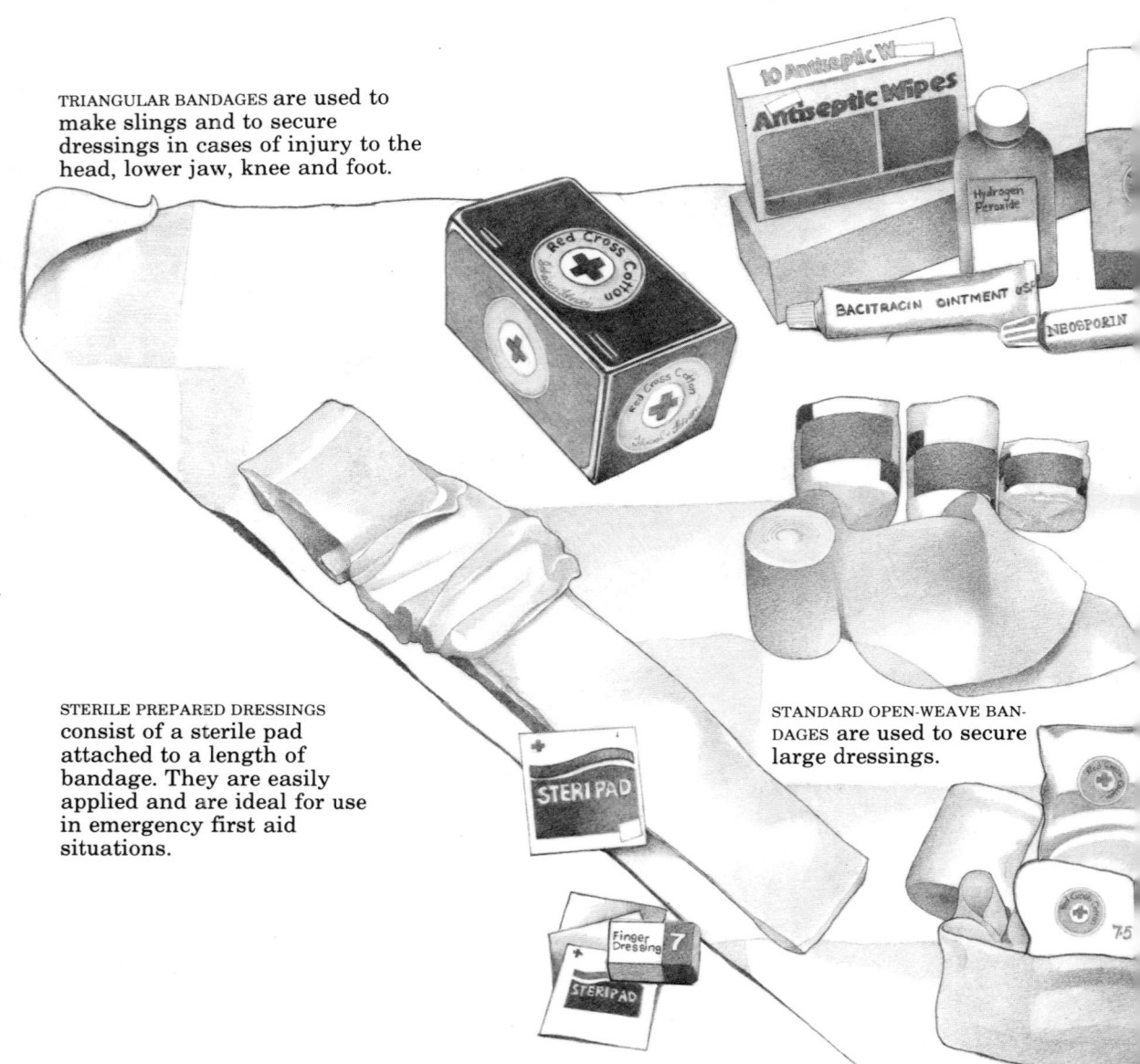

TRIANGULAR BANDAGES are used to make slings and to secure dressings in cases of injury to the head, lower jaw, knee and foot.

STERILE PREPARED DRESSINGS consist of a sterile pad attached to a length of bandage. They are easily applied and are ideal for use in emergency first aid situations.

STANDARD OPEN-WEAVE BANDAGES are used to secure large dressings.

CONFORMING BANDAGES have a soft, open weave which easily accommodates awkward shapes e.g. hand or foot.

A comprehensive first aid kit is invaluable for the prompt treatment of minor accidents in the home and the wise family will insure also that a suitable smaller kit is kept in the car at all times. First aid materials should also be carried on vacation, particularly if you are camping, trailering or boating.

Made-up kits are readily available but it is simple enough to make up your own – and often more economical. The container should be clearly marked and kept easily accessible.

THE CONTAINER for a home first aid kit should be a strong metal or plastic box with a firmly-closing lid. It should be accessible – but beyond a child's reach.

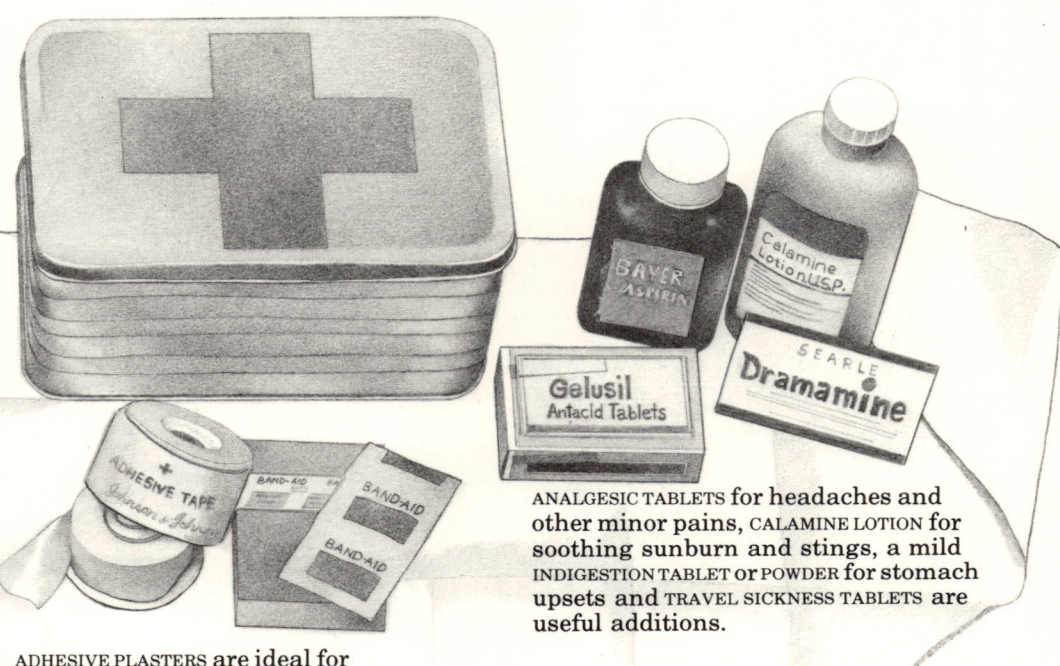

ANALGESIC TABLETS for headaches and other minor pains, CALAMINE LOTION for soothing sunburn and stings, a mild INDIGESTION TABLET or POWDER for stomach upsets and TRAVEL SICKNESS TABLETS are useful additions.

ADHESIVE PLASTERS are ideal for minor cuts and grazes. A ROLL OF ADHESIVE TAPE is also useful for securing dressings.

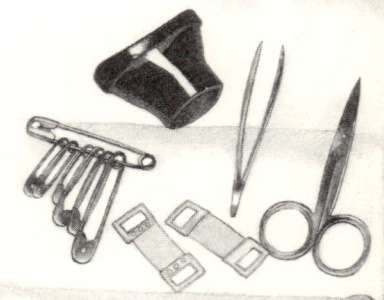

EYE-BATH, TWEEZERS, SHARP SCISSORS AND SAFETY-PINS (or BANDAGE CLIPS) should always be kept in the first aid kit.

The first aid kit

A well stocked first aid kit, adequate for the prompt treatment of most home injuries, should contain these items.

Sterile gauze and cotton
Four-by-fours and individual prepacked bandaids
2 rolled gauze bandages
2 triangular bandages
2 rolls of adhesive tape,
 (1 of 1in; 1 of ½in)
Antiseptic cream
Tincture of iodine
Calamine lotion
Aspirin tablets
Antacid tablets or liquid
Dramamine tablets or liquid
Tweezers, sharp scissors, safety-pins and thermometer

Home Cures

Never be afraid to call on your doctor for advice – it is far better to be safe than sorry – but remember that many minor illnesses may equally well be treated at home without a doctor's help. Bear in mind also that many conditions get better without any treatment.

Typically, there is no cure for the common cold; calling in the doctor will not help at all. All you can usefully do is to treat the symptoms and reduce the level of discomfort while the cold runs its course. Aspirin will relieve headache and help to bring down the temperature; the pharmacist will recommend something for the stuffy nose and will also give you something to suppress the cough and ease the sore throat.

Diarrhea is a condition which can, and should, be treated at home, at least initially. Many forms of infectious diarrhea cause excess secretion of fluid from the body, but do not hinder the absorption of fluid into it. As long as the patient isn't vomiting, he should drink as much fluid – 'clear liquid,' with sugar added – as possible. Unless the patient has severe cramps, an antispasmodic (prescribed by a doctor) can be useful. If diarrhea persists for more than two days, is accompanied by fever, or by blood in the feces, you should consult a doctor. Wash all utensils after use and wash your hands thoroughly after using the toilet.

Antacids are simple remedies for indigestion but, if the condition persists, ask your doctor for advice. The same antacids should be tried to control vomiting, although a prolonged bout does require the attention of a doctor.

Toothache or earache may be alleviated by painkillers such as aspirin or acetominophen in recommended dosages, but, if earache persists for more than a day, ask the doctor's advice without further delay.

In the case of a nosebleed, lean forward and pinch the outside of the offending nostril against the dividing wall inside the nose; a cold pack on the back of the neck may help. If bleeding has not stopped within about ten minutes, plug the nostril with cotton. Nearly all nosebleeds stop by themselves and only if the blood loss exceeds half a pint should the doctor be called.

Never prick a boil – you will only spread the infection. Keep the surrounding skin clean and dry. If the boil bursts, clean the area carefully with an antiseptic, using a sterile swab or cotton ball or clean tissue, and cover with a dry dressing.

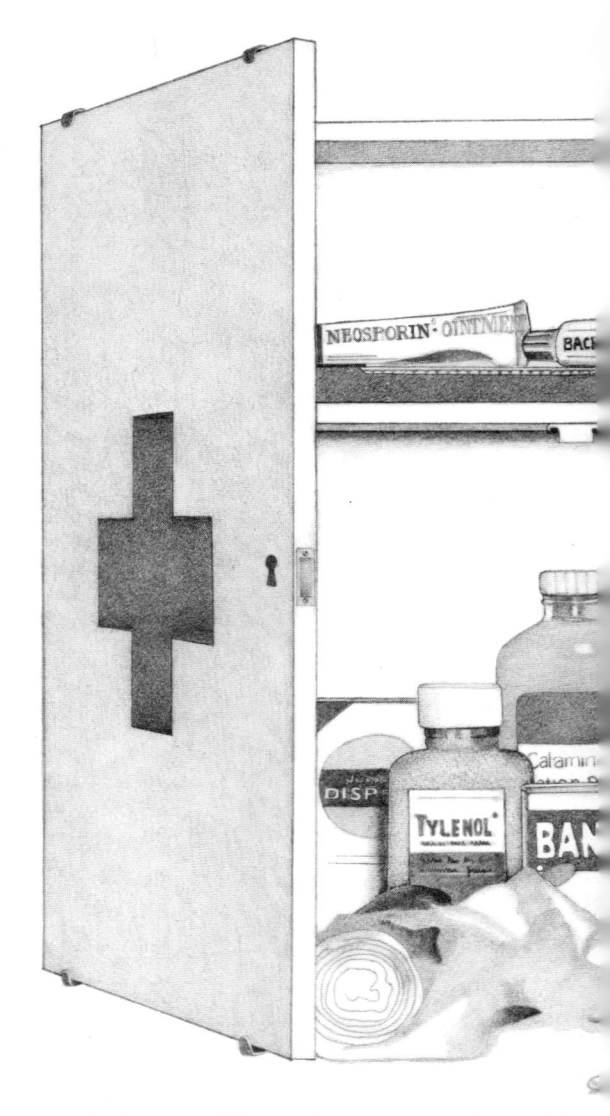

Every prudent family keeps a medicine cabinet – safely away from children – but never keep old medicines left over after a treatment prescribed by your doctor has been completed.

The home medicine chest should contain a selection of bandages and adhesive plaster dressings for wounds, plus cotton and gauze for cleansing wounds and an eyebath which may be used with warm water to wash grit from the eye.

Medicines should include soluble aspirin

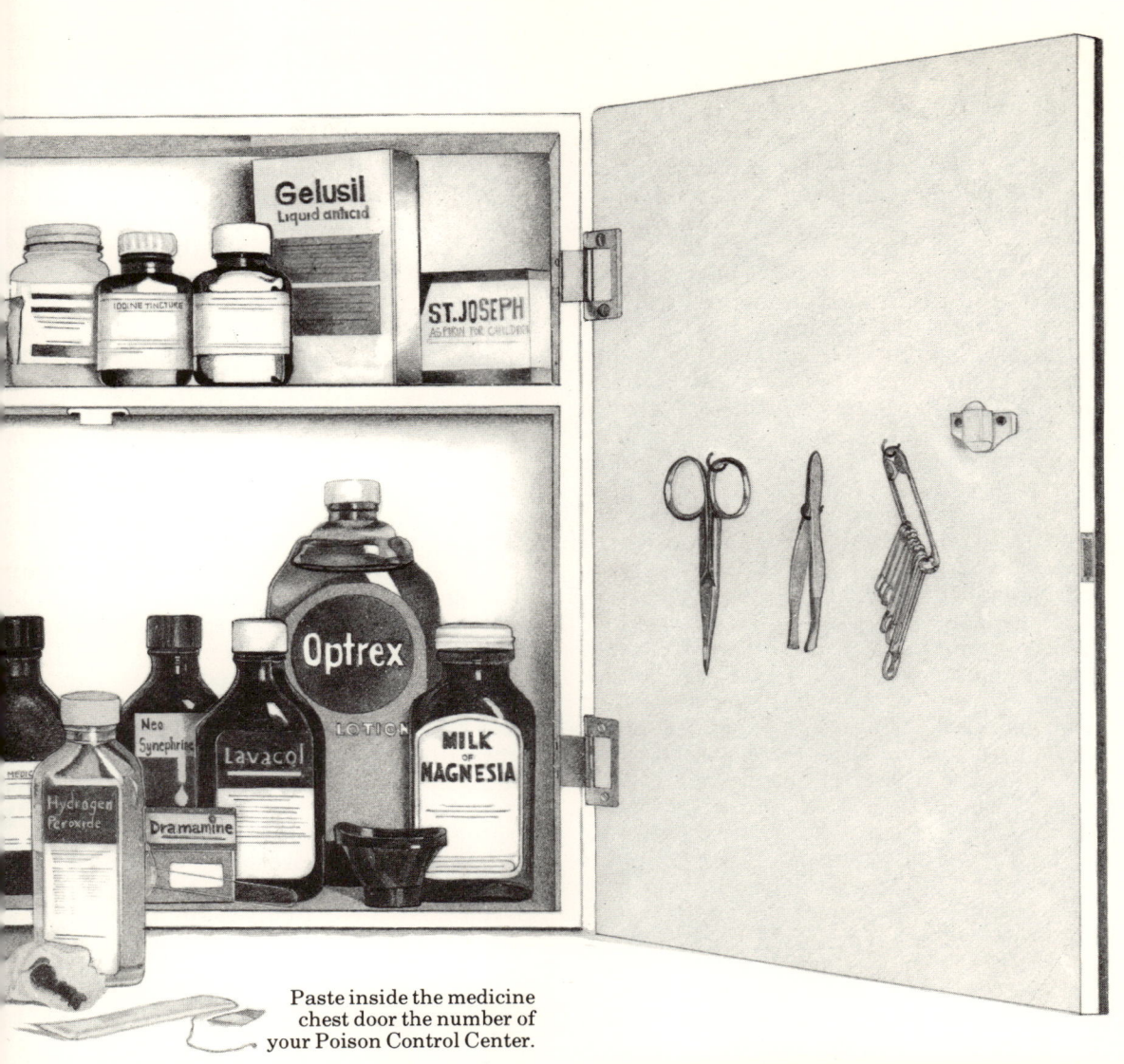

Paste inside the medicine chest door the number of your Poison Control Center.

or acetominophen and junior aspirin if there are children in the family. Antacid tablets or bicarbonate of soda will help indigestion and vomiting. Travel sickness tablets are often useful and so is a mixture for alleviating diarrhea. Do not keep laxatives; an occasional bout of constipation is not harmful, but if it persists consult your doctor.

Calamine lotion will relieve sunburn and help itching insect bites, for which an alternative is an antibacterial cream. An antiseptic cream and a liquid antiseptic should also be kept for cleansing wounds.

Always remember that, if a patient is not within the scope of home care, or worsens in spite of it, or if there is any uncertainty, consult your doctor without delay.

The medicine cabinet

DRESSINGS: a selection of adhesive plasters, gauze and bandages.
CLEANSING MATERIALS: cotton, sterile swabs, antiseptic liquid.
PAIN KILLERS: aspirin (including 'junior' aspirin), and acetominophen.
MEDICINES: proprietary mixtures for treatment of diarrhea, indigestion, sickness; plus prescribed medicines.
CREAMS: proprietary brand antiseptic creams, tincture of iodine.
THERMOMETER, SCISSORS, PINS.

The Fire Risk

Of all domestic hazards, that of fire is the most serious. A minor flare-up in a frying pan, an incorrectly wired plug on a new electrical appliance, even a cigarette left smouldering on the edge of an ash-try, can rapidly develop into a raging blaze.

In order to burn, a fire needs heat, fuel and oxygen and all fire extinguishers work on the principle of removing one of these elements. Gas fire extinguishers are filled with a heavy inert gas, usually carbon dioxide or carbon tetrachloride, which will blanket the flames and starve them of oxygen. Because the gas does not conduct electricity, they are ideal for electrical fires.

Water is the most commonly used substance and is suitable for most fires with the exception of those involving live electrical equipment or burning liquids. When the water hits the fire, it vaporizes, cutting off the air supply and, simultaneously, reducing the temperature of the material on fire. Water extinguishers must *never* be used on electrical fires: water is a good conductor and the user could receive a severe or even fatal shock. Foam extinguishers form a dense blanket over the burning material which cuts off the air supply. They are safe for use with all types of fire but are particularly effective against burning liquids such as gasoline, oils and paints.

It is useful to keep a small gas, foam or powder extinguisher in the kitchen, to kill fat or electrical fires, while a water-filled extinguisher may be positioned near the middle of the house so that it can quickly be taken to any room.

Children and the elderly are particularly at risk from clothing catching fire if the house has open fires or uses electric-bar radiators. Guard all fires thoroughly and, wherever possible, choose fire-resistant materials for children's nightclothes.

If someone's clothing does catch fire, knock them to the ground immediately so that the rising flames cannot engulf the head. Smother the flames with a woollen coat or blanket and summon an ambulance immediately. While waiting for help to arrive, give treatment for BURNS (ACTION DETAILS **pp 86-7**) and SHOCK (ACTION DETAILS **pp 90-91**).

If a serious fire does break out, *do not* wait to rescue possessions, however valuable. Evacuate the house immediately and make sure that everyone is accounted for. If you have to search smoke-filled rooms, say for a child who may have become trapped, cover your face with a wet cloth to protect your lungs from the heat and smoke. As you leave the building, close all doors behind you; open doors and windows increase the draft and accelerate the fire's progress.

Only when you are sure everyone is safe should you try to tackle the fire and then only if you have a clear exit route: *take no risks* of becoming cut off or lost in the smoke.

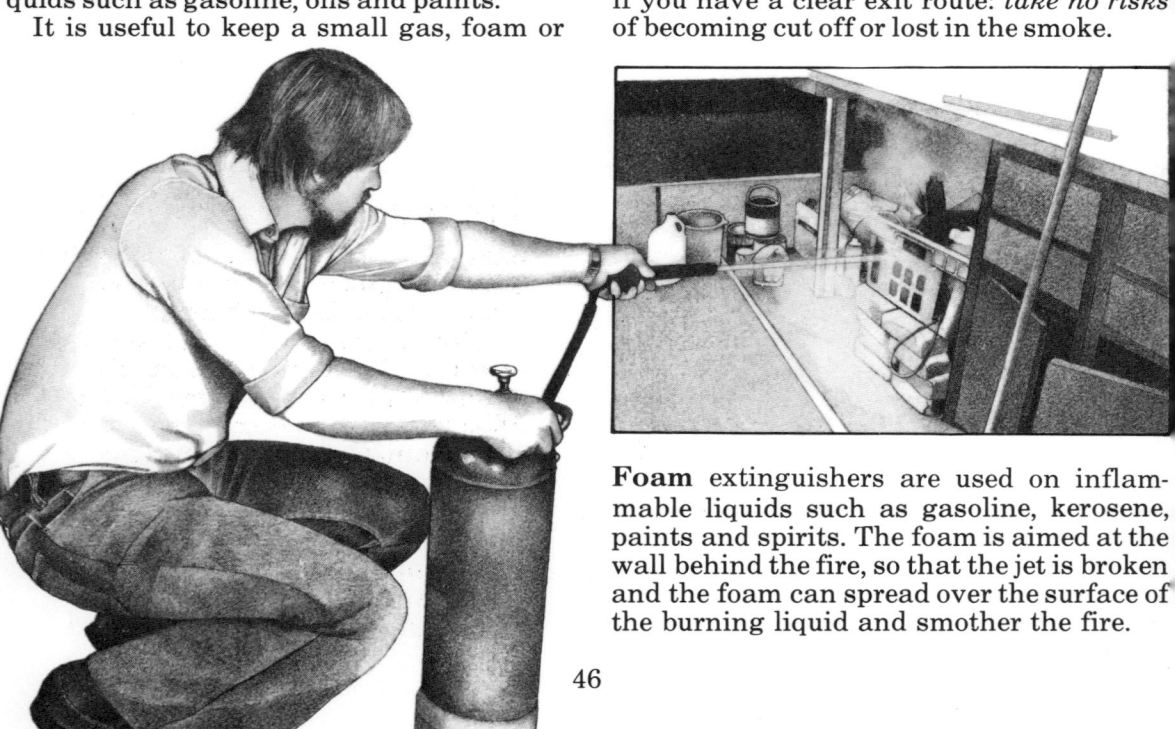

Foam extinguishers are used on inflammable liquids such as gasoline, kerosene, paints and spirits. The foam is aimed at the wall behind the fire, so that the jet is broken and the foam can spread over the surface of the burning liquid and smother the fire.

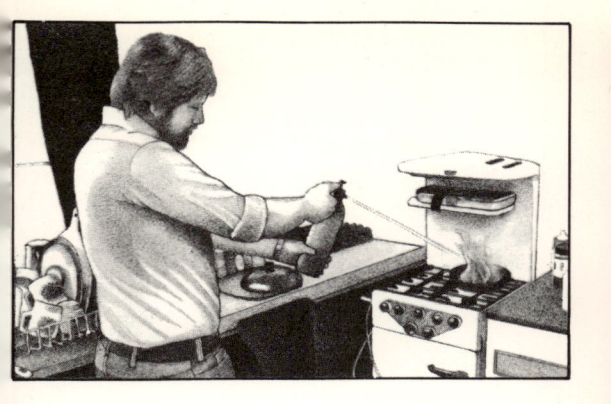

Dry powder extinguishers are ideal for frying-pan fires where it is essential that the fat is extinguished quickly. If an extinguisher is not available, smother the flames with a close-fitting lid or a damp towel *and leave the pan to cool*: very hot fat may flare up again on contact with air.

When fire is discovered

1 Evacuate the house quickly
2 Check all persons accounted for
3 Raise the alarm immediately
4 Tackle fire if safe to do so

If someone's clothing is alight

1 Knock them to the ground
2 Smother the flames
3 Summon an ambulance immediately
4 Treat for burns and shock

If trapped by fire

1 Close doors and windows
2 Block edges of doors with coats
3 Call for help from window

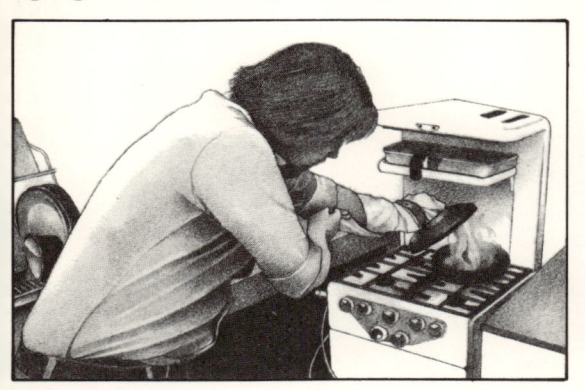

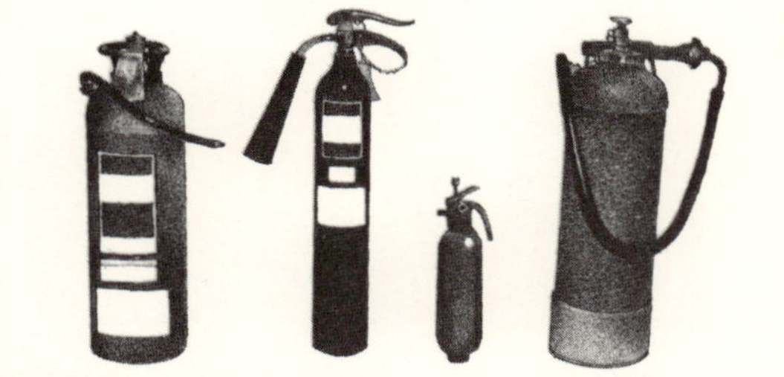

The main types of extinguisher suitable for domestic, office and workshop use – water, carbon dioxide, dry powder and foam.

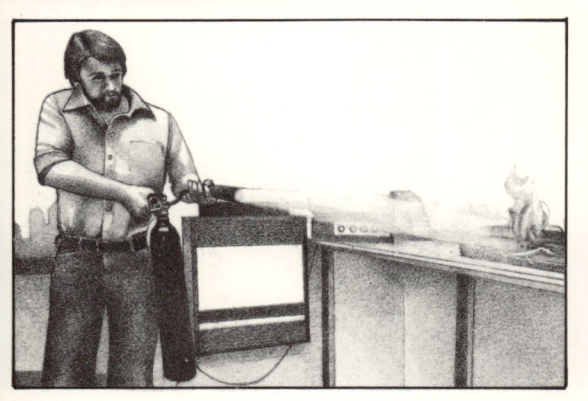

Carbon dioxide extinguishers are for use on electrical fires and small amounts of burning liquids. In electrical equipment the jet is aimed directly at the fire; in liquids, at the near edge – driving the fire back with a sweeping motion of the horn.

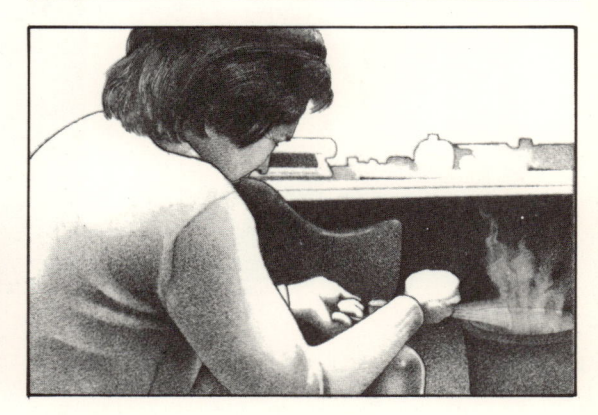

Water-filled extinguishers are suitable for all fires except those involving live electrical equipment or inflammable liquid. The jet is directed at the base of the fire and is swept back and forth across the fire until all flames are quenched.

ACCIDENT ACTION

Action Priorities

Most of the accidents occurring in the home involve relatively minor cuts and bruises, burns, foreign bodies blown into the eye and occasional insect bites. Their treatment is simple and will be found in the relevant sections of this book. Most will heal quickly and only in cases of persistent pain or obvious infection will medical attention be necessary.

It is, however, in the event of a more serious accident that the well-informed first aider can prove invaluable. The interval between the accident happening and the arrival of the emergency services is vital. *Prompt action can save a life.*

☐ **Keep calm, take charge, organize**
Enlist help if possible to . . .

☎ *Telephone for an ambulance and, if necessary, police and rescue services*

Keep bystanders away from danger
Control traffic flow
Extinguish, or at least contain, fires
Comfort and reassure those involved but not requiring immediate attention

☐ *Withdraw from danger*
If casualties are endangered by fire, spilt chemicals or gases, move them quickly out of danger. If there is no further immediate threat to life, treat all casualties where they are, moving them as little as possible.

☐ *Take immediate action*
Check all casualties for the following major threats to life – and act quickly.

BREATHING STOPPED OR FAILING	52/57
CHOKING	54
HEART STOPPED	58/59
SEVERE BLEEDING	62/69

☐ Then check each casualty for further, but non-critical, injuries

UNCONSCIOUSNESS	70/71
BROKEN BONES	72/83
BURNS AND SCALDS	86/87
SEVERE SHOCK	90/91

☐ *Do not*
Try to be sophisticated: improvise where necessary. Shirts, handkerchiefs, towels and any other clean cloth will serve as a dressing. Ties and belts make perfectly adequate emergency slings. A stocking or scarf will hold a dressing in place in the absence of a bandage.

☐ *Do not*
Give the casualty anything to eat or drink, except in the case of a conscious burn victim in which case moisten his lips regularly with a wet cloth.

☐ *Do not*
Overheat a casualty: he should be kept warm but one coat or blanket will be quite sufficient.

☐ *Gather as much information as possible*
The more information you can pass on to doctors and ambulance crew, the more effectively they can operate.

Breathing Stopped

Many different factors may cause breathing difficulties, or cause the breathing to stop completely, but they can be grouped into two main categories.

1 Obstruction of the breathing passages
☐ by water or smoke or by food or vomit becoming lodged in the windpipe. Some foreign bodies can not only cause a direct blockage themselves but may also cause muscular spasm of the respiratory tract which may obstruct the passage of air to the lungs
☐ by the tongue falling to the back of the throat if an unconscious victim is lying on his back
☐ by compression of the windpipe through strangulation or throttling
☐ by suffocation, by blocking of the nose and mouth *e.g.* by a plastic bag
☐ by damage to the inside of the throat due to scalding or insect stings or through swallowing a corrosive liquid

2 Interference with breathing mechanism
☐ by crushing of the chest, for example in a crowd incident or in the severe impact of an automobile accident
☐ by direct effect on the nerves in the brain which control breathing – as may happen in electric shock, poisoning by some industrial gases and pesticides, or through taking an overdose of drugs, such as barbiturates, morphine or aspirin.
☐ by disease such as polio, or through an injury to the spine, either of which may interfere with the nerves controlling the breathing mechanism

☐ by prevention of the body's use of its oxygen supply – as in poisoning by some gases or choking by smoke

Whatever the cause, swift action is required if a life is to be saved and lasting damage is to be avoided.

☎ *Summon expert help and start artificial respiration at once*

Action details

It is essential that the victim has a clear airway so first clear any fluid, debris or vomit from the mouth and bend the head back as far as possible, pressing the top of the head down and back with one hand while holding up the chin with the other. This will move the tongue forward, opening up the breathing passages.

This may be all that is necessary for breathing to restart spontaneously and if this is the case, move the casualty into the RECOVERY POSITION (**below and on pp 70-71**). However, keep a very careful watch on the casualty's condition; he may be sick, in which case clear the mouth again immediately to remove the danger of choking, or his breathing may falter or fail completely, in which case immediate action is required.

If breathing does *not* restart once the breathing passages are open, or if it fails while the casualty is in the recovery position, ARTIFICIAL RESPIRATION (ACTION DETAILS **pp 52-7**) must be started at once. Use mouth-to-mouth resuscitation or one of the manual methods described below.

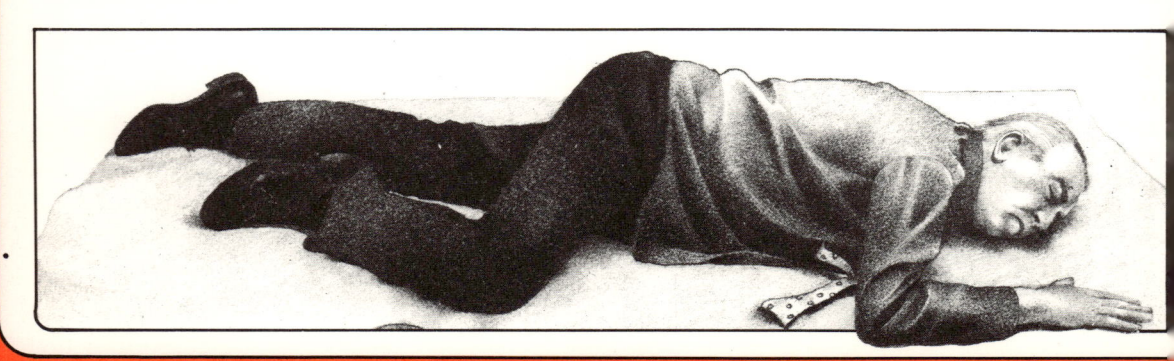

The Heimlich Maneuver

Death by choking is commonly caused by the blocking of the respiratory passage by a piece of food sucked against the larynx as the victim inhales. The lungs are therefore usually filled with air at the time of the accident and this situation is fundamental to the Heimlich Maneuver.

The rescuer stands behind the victim and reaches around to grasp one clenched fist with the free hand. The fist is held, thumb side toward the body, just above the navel and below the rib cage. A sharp inward and upward thrust into the victim's abdomen, repeated if necessary, compresses the air in the lungs and expels the food particle forcibly from the throat.

In severe cases, and especially if vomiting occurs, the casualty should be placed in the RECOVERY POSITION (**pp 70-71**) until medical attention can be summoned.

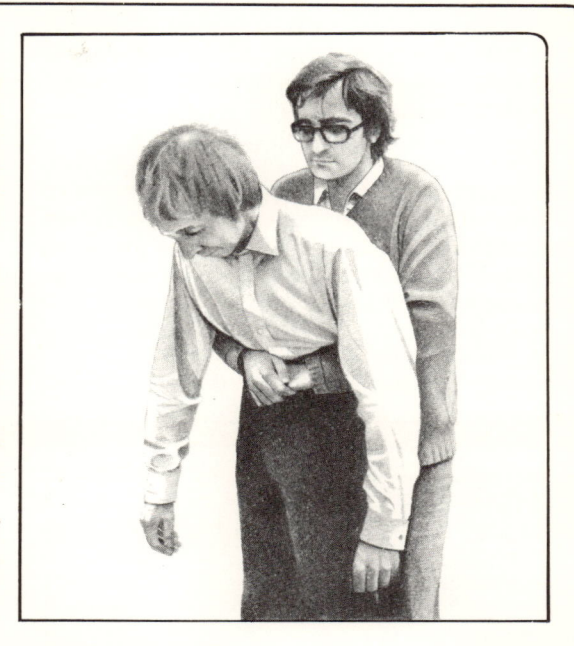

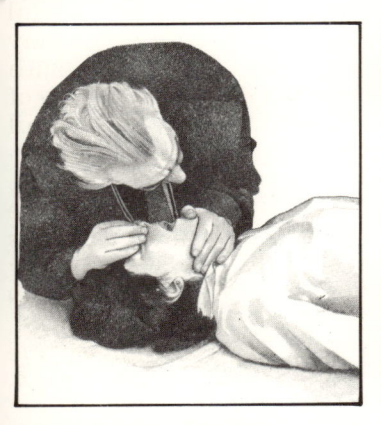

The 'Kiss of Life' 52-3
The mouth-to-mouth method of artificial respiration is the most effective known and should be used whenever possible. However, if the casualty has suffered facial damage, use one of the alternative (manual) techniques described on pp 54-7.

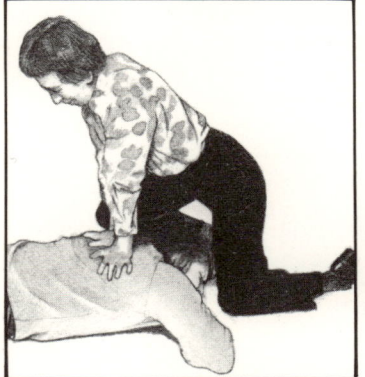

Holger-Nielsen 54-5
Probably the best-known of the manual techniques and very effective in cases of drowning as, having the casualty in a face-down position, it allows very free drainage of water from the mouth.

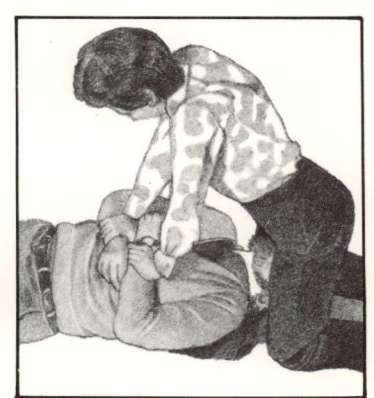

Sylvester 56-7
An excellent alternative to mouth-to-mouth resuscitation when the casualty has suffered facial damage, as the body lies face-upward. This position, like the 'kiss of life' also allows external heart massage to be performed.

Artificial Respiration

1 The first thing to do with any unconscious accident or emergency victim is to check whether or not he is breathing easily. If he is not, ARTIFICIAL RESPIRATION should be started without delay. Seconds count – but act smoothly.

2 Ensure that the victim has a clear airway. Clear the mouth of fluids or obstructions and tilt the head well back as shown. This will move the tongue forward, opening up the air passages.

☎ *Telephone for a doctor or ambulance without delay*

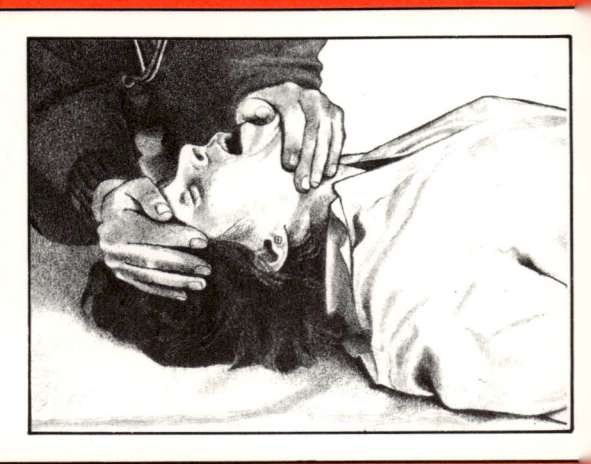

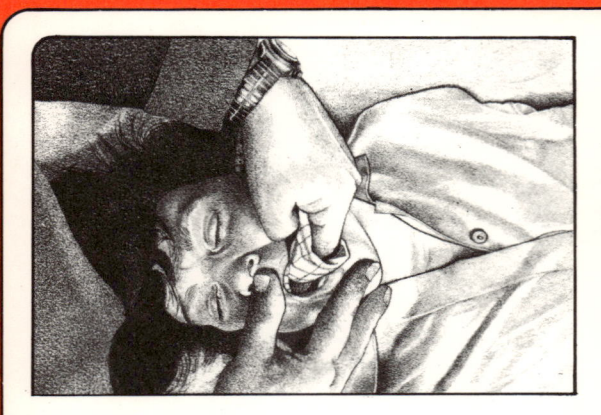

Artificial respiration

1 If breathing does *not* restart, turn the victim on his back, open his mouth and remove any obstructing mud or vomit. Cup one hand beneath the neck, lift slightly and support the head in this position. Place the other hand on the forehead so that the forefinger and thumb can reach the nose.

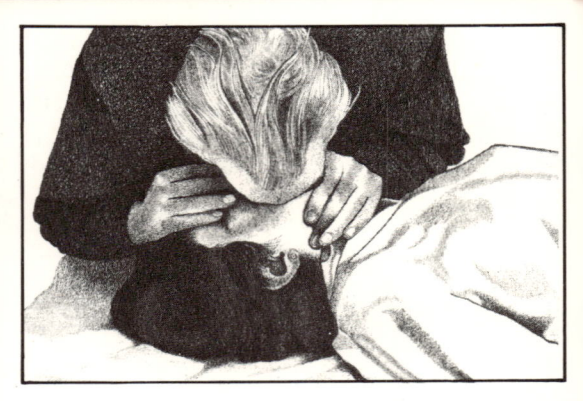

2 Pinching the nose closed with one hand and cupping the chin in the other, take a deep breath and then seal your lips about the victim's open mouth. Blow steadily into his lungs, making the chest rise. If it does not, you probably have not got the head tilted far enough back, or the throat may be blocked. In the latter case roll the victim over and hit his back.

How long should artificial respiration be continued?

The answer is, until the patient begins to breathe easily again. But even then be ready to start again if he gets into difficulties. Otherwise, carry on for as long as possible, taking turns if others are present. Do not stop until expert help arrives or until a doctor declares the casualty dead.

If the casualty's heart stops then EXTERNAL HEART MASSAGE (ACTION DETAILS **pp 58-9**) should be alternated with artificial respiration. However, while artificial respiration may be started if breath-

The 'Kiss of Life'

3 The recovery position (See also pages 70-71)

Stage 2 may be all that is necessary for breathing to start again spontaneously. If it does so, place the patient in the recovery position but watch him carefully.

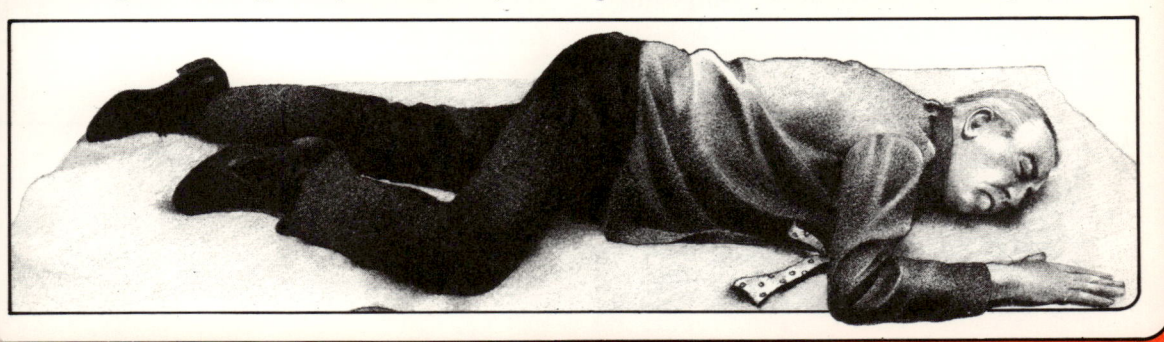

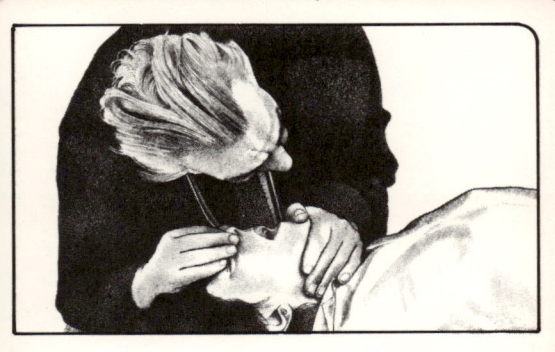

3 Remove your mouth and let the chest deflate naturally as you take your next deep breath. Repeat the sequence. The first four or five inflations should be rapid, to saturate the patient's blood with oxygen, but after that you can settle to a steady rhythm in pace with your own breathing. Do not blow too hard; just hard enough to produce a natural rise in the casualty's chest. Keep checking the strength of the carotid pulse in the side of the neck.

For small children

Cover both nose and mouth with your own mouth and blow *gently* so as not to cause damage to the sensitive tissue of the child's lungs.

With an adult casualty whose mouth cannot be opened, or who has a mouth injury, seal your lips around the nose only and use the hand beneath the chin to keep his mouth firmly closed during each inflation of the lungs.

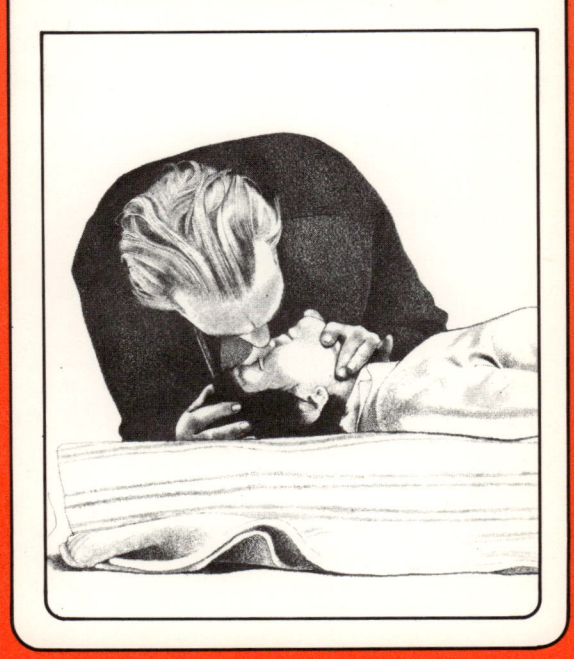

ing appears to be failing, heart massage should never be used unless the heart has definitely stopped beating.

Mouth-to-mouth resuscitation is the most efficient method of artificial respiration but alternative methods, for use in certain situations, are described on the following four pages.

Artificial Respiration

Although mouth-to-mouth resuscitation is the most effective method of artificial respiration it is sometimes not practical due to the presence of severe facial injury or fracture of the jaw. In such cases either the HOLGER-NIELSEN METHOD (**these pages**) or the SYLVESTER METHOD (**see pp 56-7**) should be used. Both are manual methods of manipulating the upper body to expand and contract the casualty's chest.

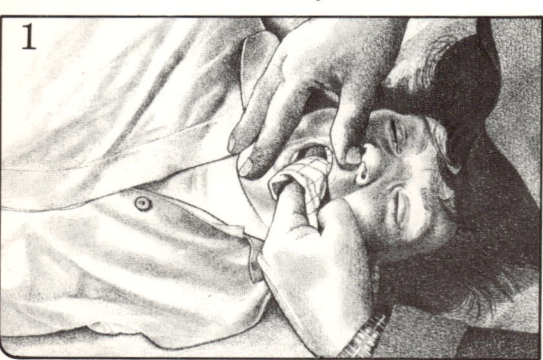

Action details

Quickly clear the mouth of any obstruction (1) and roll the casualty onto his front. Arrange the hands to form a cushion for the head which should be turned to the side and slightly downward. Kneel at the casualty

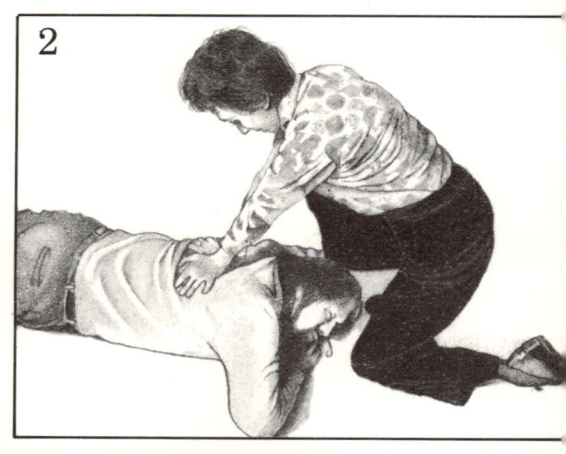

Drowning

In the case of a casualty pulled from the water unconscious, *do not* make any attempt to force water from the lungs or stomach. To do so may cause internal injury. The victim needs air urgently and properly-applied ARTIFICIAL RESPIRATION will make air bubble past any watery obstruction to reach the lungs.

Action details

1 Begin mouth-to-mouth resuscitation without delay, taking turns if others are there to help.

☎ ***Get someone to telephone for an ambulance at once***

2 Continue artificial respiration until expert help arrives or until a doctor declares the casualty dead.

3 EXTERNAL HEART COMPRESSION (ACTION DETAILS **pp 58-9**) may be needed if the heart has stopped but this should only be done on a firm surface.

Choking

If the victim is coughing, allow him to continue but keep a close watch on his condition. If the offending object is firmly lodged in the throat or windpipe swift action is needed. Give three or four sharp blows between the shoulder blades to dislodge the obstruction.

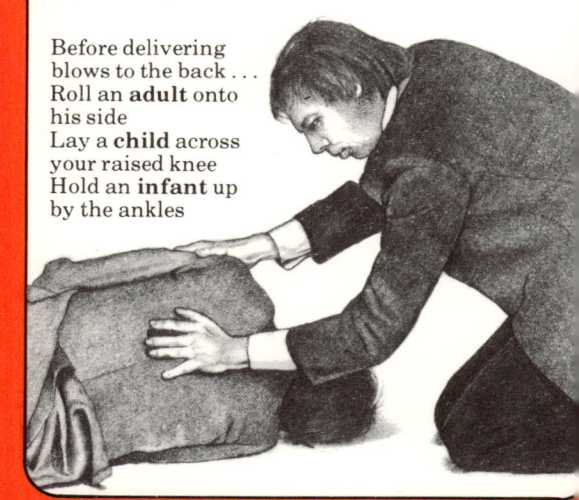

Before delivering blows to the back...
Roll an **adult** onto his side
Lay a **child** across your raised knee
Hold an **infant** up by the ankles

Holger-Nielsen Method 54/55

...ad (2) and place the hands, thumbs touching, just below the shoulder blades. With the ...ms straight, rock forward (3) to force the air ...om the casualty's lungs. Rock back (4) ...oothly raising the casualty's elbows to ...pand his chest and draw air into his lungs. ...peat 12 times per minute.

DO NOT jerk the arms or pause too long at stage 4. Aim to establish a smooth, steady rhythm in time with your own natural rate of breathing.

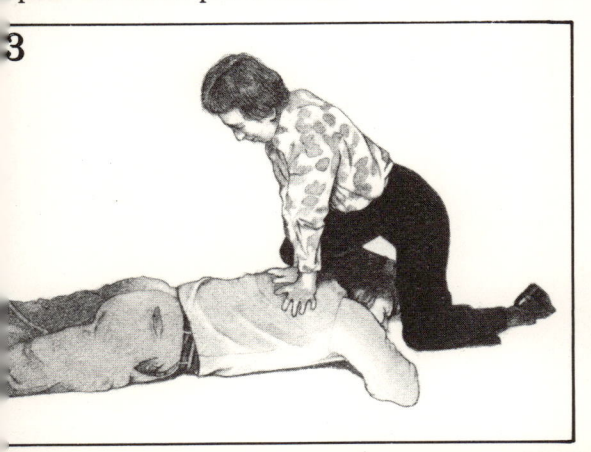

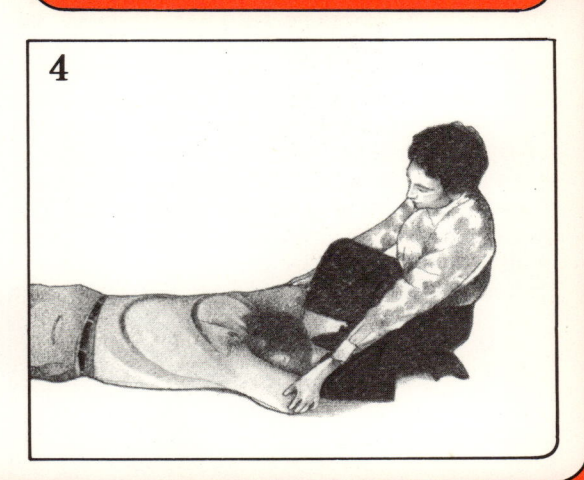

Victim overcome by gas or smoke

Before entering a gas-filled room, first take several deep breaths to saturate the blood with oxygen. Then go in quickly, holding your breath and wearing a lifeline if at all possible, and drag the victim to safety. If he is trapped, try and turn off the gas (or car engine), open doors and windows and leave quickly. Go in again as soon as the gas has dispersed. Give the victim ARTIFICIAL RESPIRATION (ACTION DETAILS pp 52-7) and summon expert help as quickly as possible. With smoke, wrap a wet cloth around your face and keep low; there is often less smoke at floor level. Grasp the victim under the arms and drag him to safety.

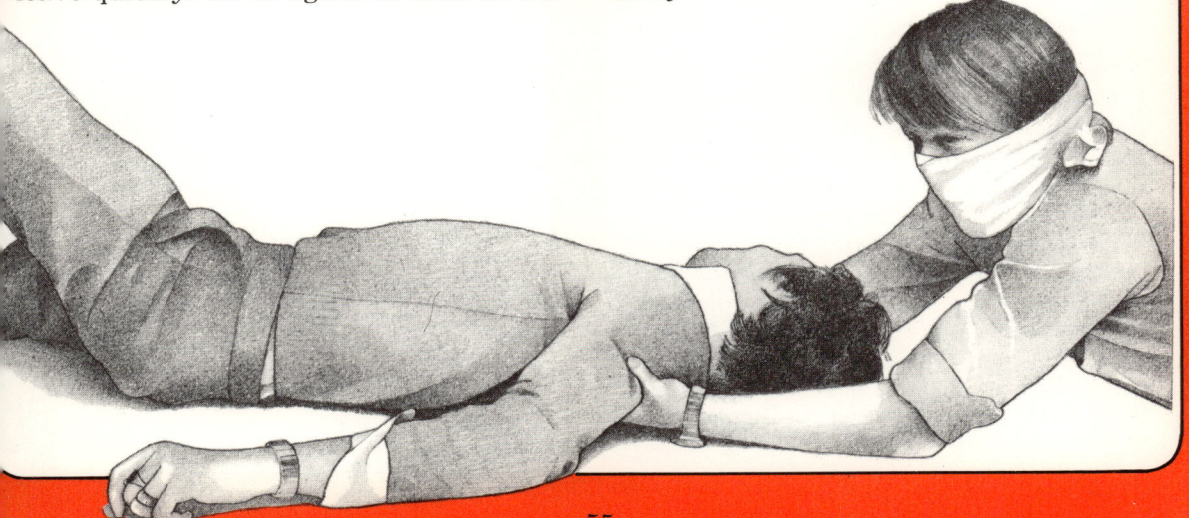

Artificial Respiration

The method of artificial respiration used will vary with the circumstances of the accident. MOUTH-TO-MOUTH RESUSCITATION (ACTION DETAILS **pp 52-3**) should always be the first choice: it is very efficient and has the advantage of allowing EXTERNAL HEART COMPRESSION (ACTION DETAILS **pp 58-9**) to be performed at the same time. HOLGER-NIELSEN is a good alternative method and is particularly useful in cases of drowning as it allows free drainage of fluids from the mouth. A third method, SYLVESTER, is a useful alternative where facial damage has occurred and, like the mouth-to-mouth method, it allows heart compression.

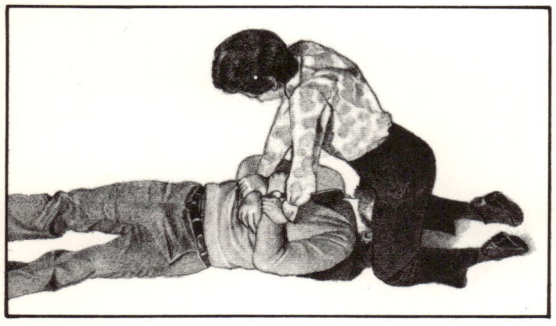

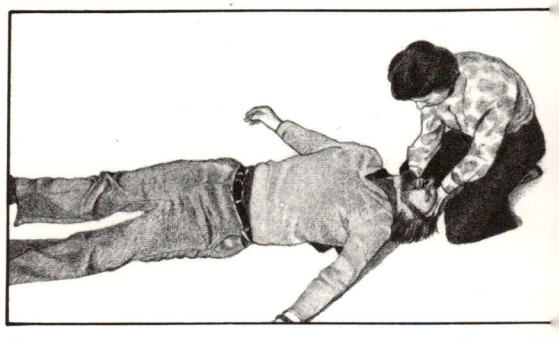

1 Lay the victim on his back on a hard surface and place a folded coat or blanket under the shoulders so that the head is tilted right back. Clear the mouth of obstructions.

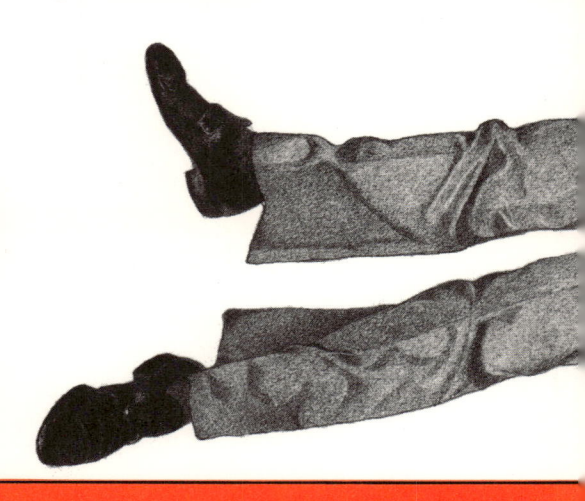

3 Rock forward until your arms are vertical. There is no need to press; the weight of your body will depress the chest wall far enough to expell air from the lungs.

Electric shock

If possible, switch off the current or pull the plug from the socket. If this is not possible, pull on the insulated cable of the appliance and drag it away from the victim. Alternatively, use a non-conducting material (a chair, stick, rolled newspaper or even a folded coat) to push or pull the casualty clear of the current source. *Do not touch him yourself.* Once contact is broken, both artificial respiration and heart massage may be necessary and these should be performed *even if he appears dead.* Lives have been lost simply through emergency action not being continued long enough.

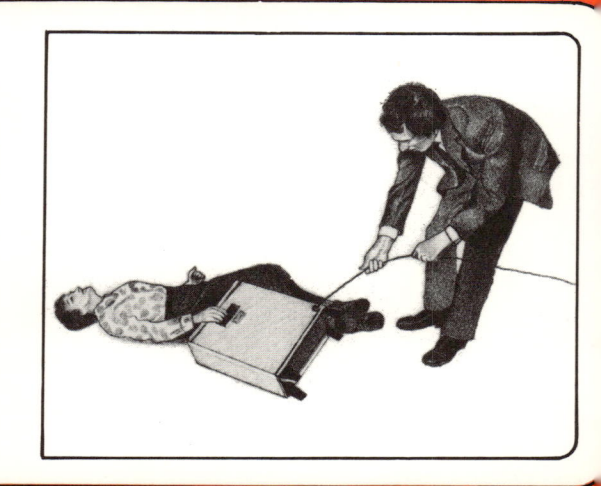

Sylvester Method 56/57

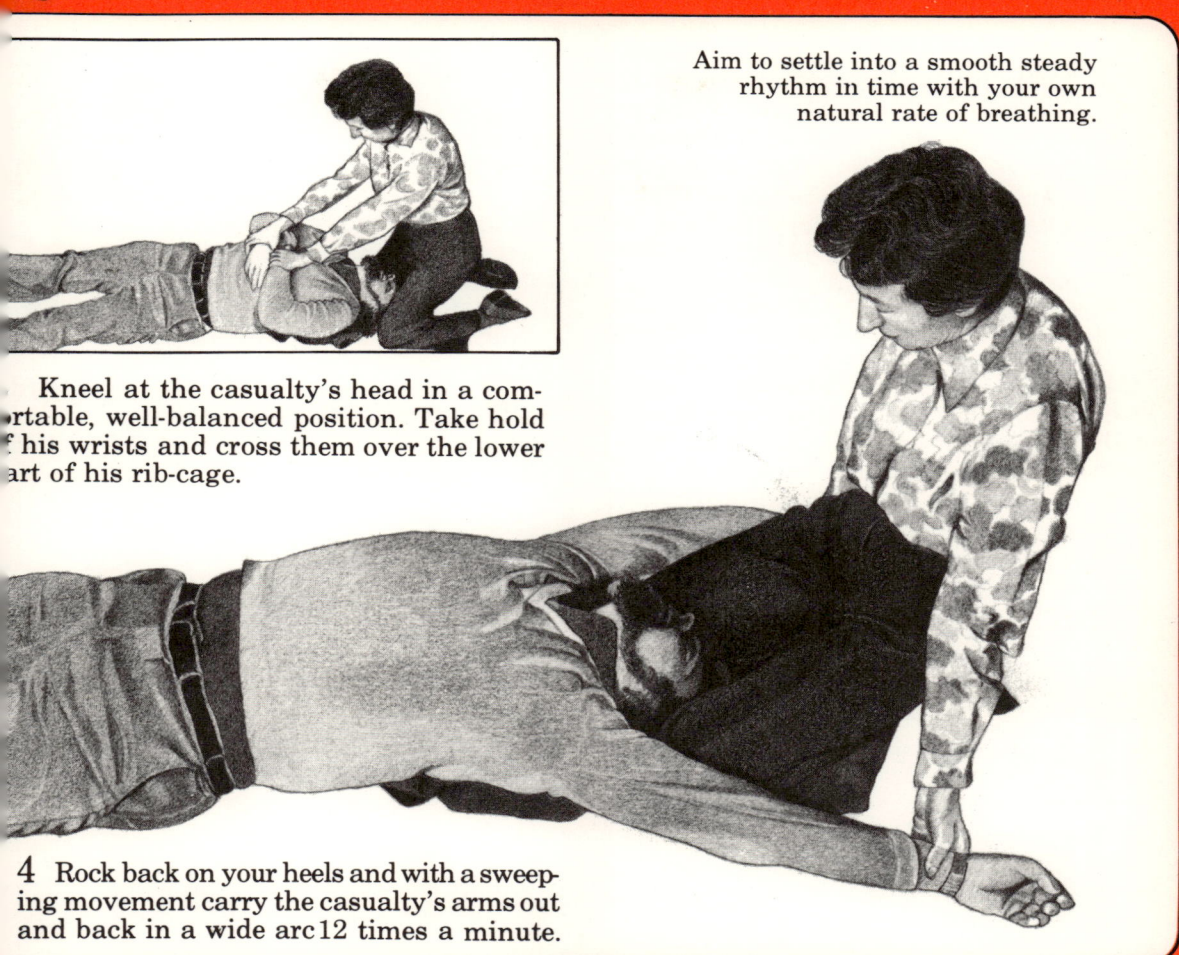

Kneel at the casualty's head in a comfortable, well-balanced position. Take hold of his wrists and cross them over the lower part of his rib-cage.

Aim to settle into a smooth steady rhythm in time with your own natural rate of breathing.

4 Rock back on your heels and with a sweeping movement carry the casualty's arms out and back in a wide arc 12 times a minute.

High-voltage shock

If the victim is in contact with high-tension cables, electric train conductor rails or high-voltage power lines, *do not approach or attempt to move him*. Alert the authorities and stay at least 50 feet away until the current has been switched off.

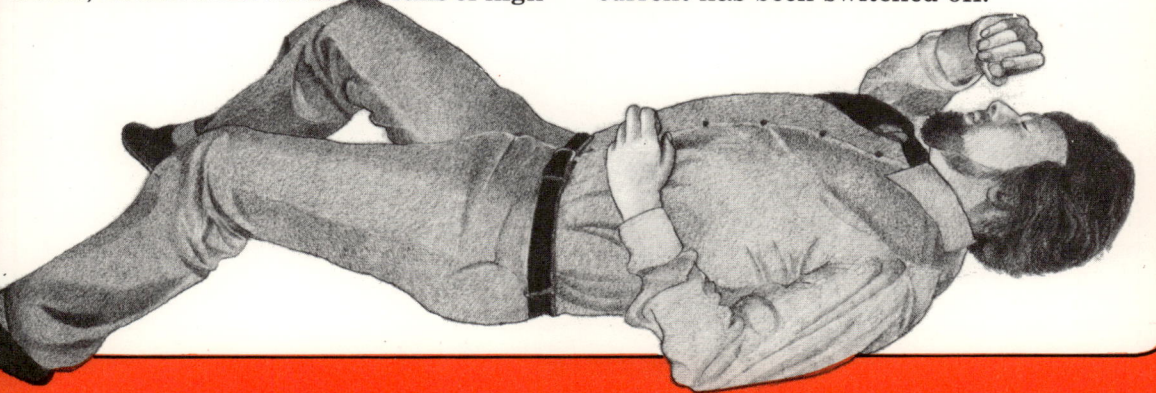

Heart Stopped

After a serious accident or other emergency not only may the victim's breathing cease but his heart may stop as well. Immediate action is necessary if his life is to be saved and if permanent physical or mental damage is to be avoided. The absolute priority is to restart the blood supply to the brain without delay: starved of oxygen for more than about 4 minutes, the brain suffers irreversible damage.

Signs and symptoms
☐ his color will be, or will become, a deathly blue-gray
☐ the pupils of the eyes will become widely dilated
☐ no pulse will be felt in either of the carotid arteries in the neck. The pulse can normally be felt by placing the fingers on the neck just above the level of the Adam's apple

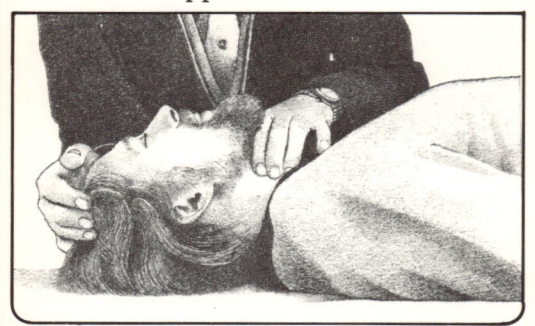

Action
Lay the casualty on his back on a firm surface – the floor or the ground. Give ONE firm blow with the edge of the hand on the lower left part of the breastbone. If this fails to restart the heart, EXTERNAL HEART MASSAGE will be needed (ACTION DETAILS **facing page**), but this should *never* be used unless you are sure that the heart is not beating.

☎ *Telephone for an ambulance as quickly as possible*

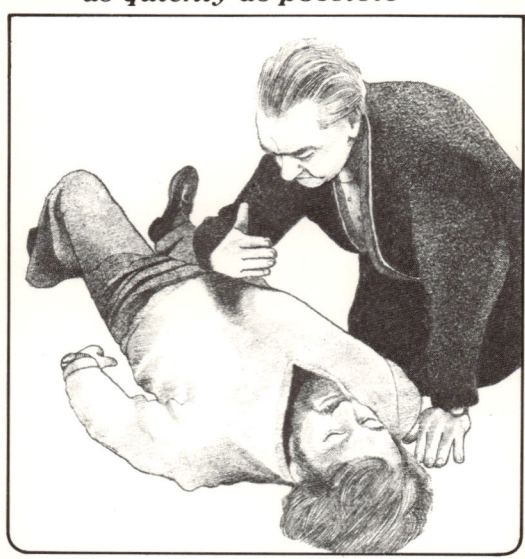

The heart and lungs
Oxygen-enriched blood is pumped from the left side of the heart into the major arteries and thence through the branching network of blood vessels to all parts of the body. Blood depleted of its oxygen by the muscles and other organs is returned to the heart and then pumped to the lungs where waste carbon dioxide is released and the blood is recharged with oxygen. This remarkable muscle contracts some 70 to 80 times a minute throughout man's life.

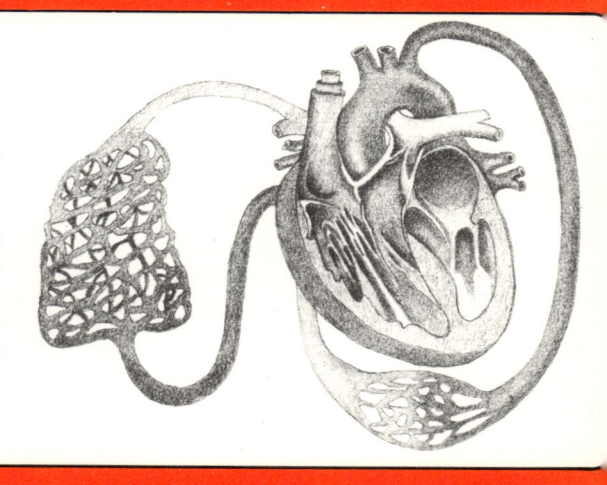

External heart compression
Kneel by the victim and place the heel of one hand on the lower half of the breastbone – keeping the fingers raised off the chest. Place the heel of the other hand on top of the first. Then, keeping the arms straight, rock forward to depress the chest wall, and back.

Adults
With an unconscious adult the chest wall will depress about 1½ inches (4 cm). Repeat 60 times per minute.

Children
The child's chest is vulnerable to rough treatment. Use *one hand only* and depress 80 times per minute.

Babies
Pressure from *two fingers only* should be used. Depress 100 times per minute.

Signs of success
Successful heart massage brings
☐ an improvement in the victim's color
☐ reduction in the size of the pupils
☐ return of the carotid pulse

Restarting respiration
Whenever the heart stops, breathing fails as well so ARTIFICIAL RESPIRATION is required in addition to heart massage, (ACTION DETAILS **pp 52-7**).

WHEN ALONE give 2 inflations of the lungs followed by 15 heart compressions. Move smoothly and quickly from one procedure to the other and back.

WHEN THERE ARE TWO OF YOU one person should perform mouth-to-mouth resuscitation while the other takes care of the heart. *But each process should be kept separate.* Alternate 1 deep lung inflation with 5 heart compressions. The person giving the 'kiss of life' should also check the carotid pulse.

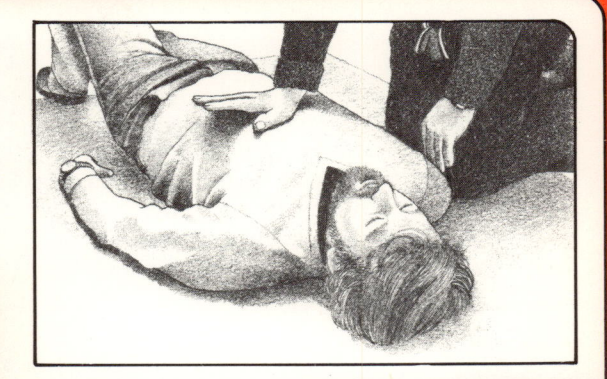

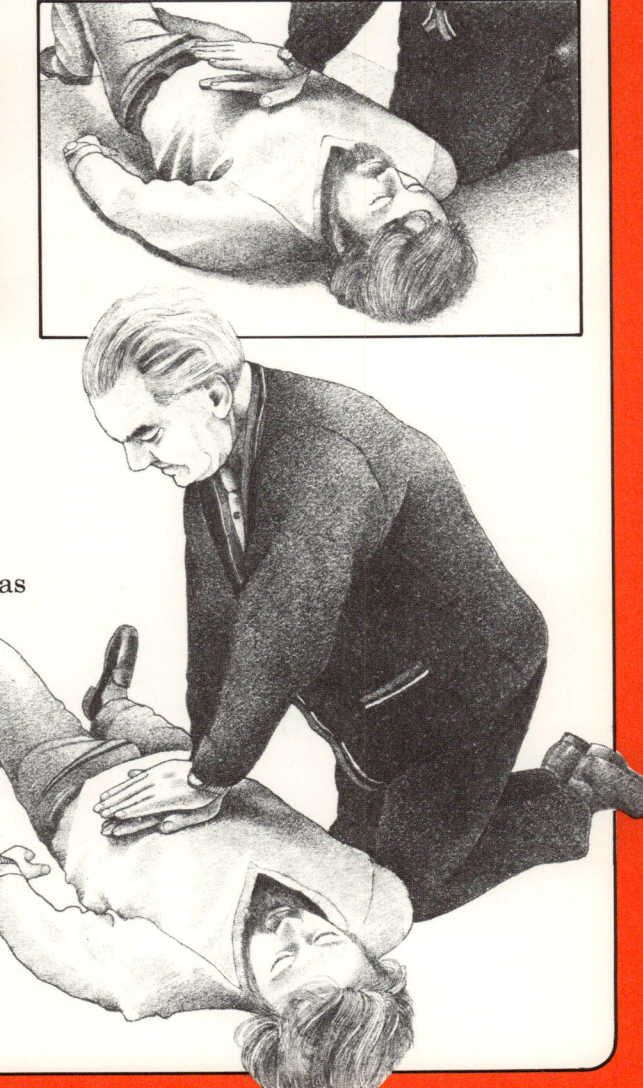

Heart Attack

Action 1

Heart attacks can be very frightening but it is important to remember that many victims do make a complete recovery and that prompt action can save a life.

The most important thing to do is to summon expert aid without delay.

☎ *Telephone for an ambulance or doctor as quickly as possible.*

Action 2

Make the sufferer comfortable but do not move him unnecessarily. Loosen tight clothing at neck, chest and waist and support him in a semi-recumbent position with a couple of pillows to raise his head and shoulders. If he is having difficulties with his breathing he should be supported in a sitting position

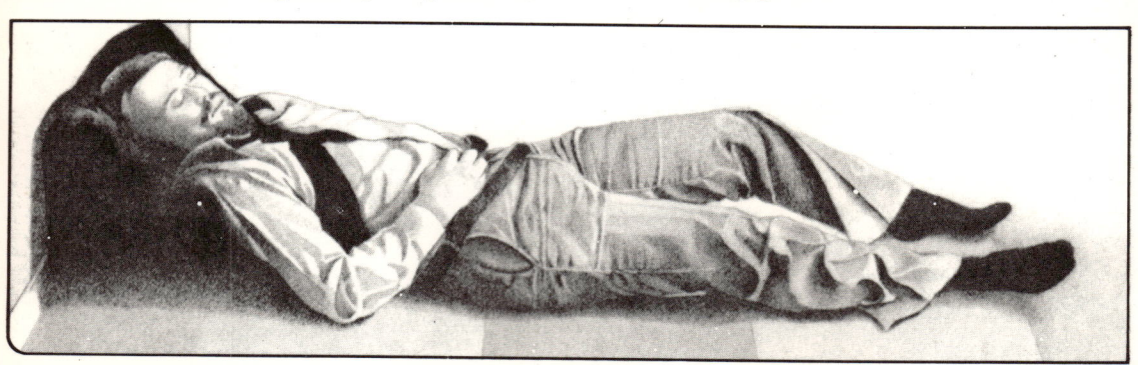

What is a heart attack?

A heart attack is the layman's term for symptoms arising from an obstruction in the supply of blood to the muscles of the heart, which means they are not getting sufficient oxygen to keep them working properly. When talking of heart attacks we normally mean coronary obstruction, or CORONARY THROMBOSIS, but another condition, ANGINA PECTORIS can produce almost identical symptoms in the patient.

As far as immediate action is concerned the precise diagnosis is immaterial; the emergency procedure to be followed is the same for both conditions.

Signs and symptoms

In CORONARY THROMBOSIS a blood clot suddenly blocks one of the arteries in the wall of the heart, cutting off the blood supply to a section of muscle. The victim experiences a vice-like pain, usually in the middle of the chest, occasionally centrally just below the rib cage. The pain often spreads to the shoulders and arms and to the throat and jaws. ANGINA occurs when the arteries supplying the heart have become narrowed so that the blood supply is inadequate. Over-exertion, excitement or shock can bring on a sudden attack of pain in the chest which often spreads to the left shoulder, arm and fingers and may affect the throat, jaws, right shoulder and upper arm as well.

In either thrombosis or angina attack the pain can be so intense that the sufferer slumps forward over a desk or chair or leans against the wall for support. A common tell-tale sign in coronary thrombosis is that the victim clutches at the centre of his chest with a tightly clenched fist and complains of it being squeezed in. In a severe attack the patient will be pale and perspiring; there may be a marked blueness about the lips, and he will have considerable difficulty breathing.

Action 3

The first two hours after a heart attack are the most dangerous so it is important to telephone for an ambulance at the first sign: a doctor may take some time to arrive at the scene.

If breathing has stopped, ARTIFICIAL RESPIRATION should be given immediately (ACTION DETAILS pp 52-7). If the heart stops, lay the victim on his back and give him *one* firm blow with the edge of your hand on the left lower part of the breastbone. If this fails to restart the heart try EXTERNAL HEART COMPRESSION (ACTION DETAILS pp 58-9). No drinks or drugs or other treatment should be given unless prescribed by a doctor. To do so could complicate the patient's condition.

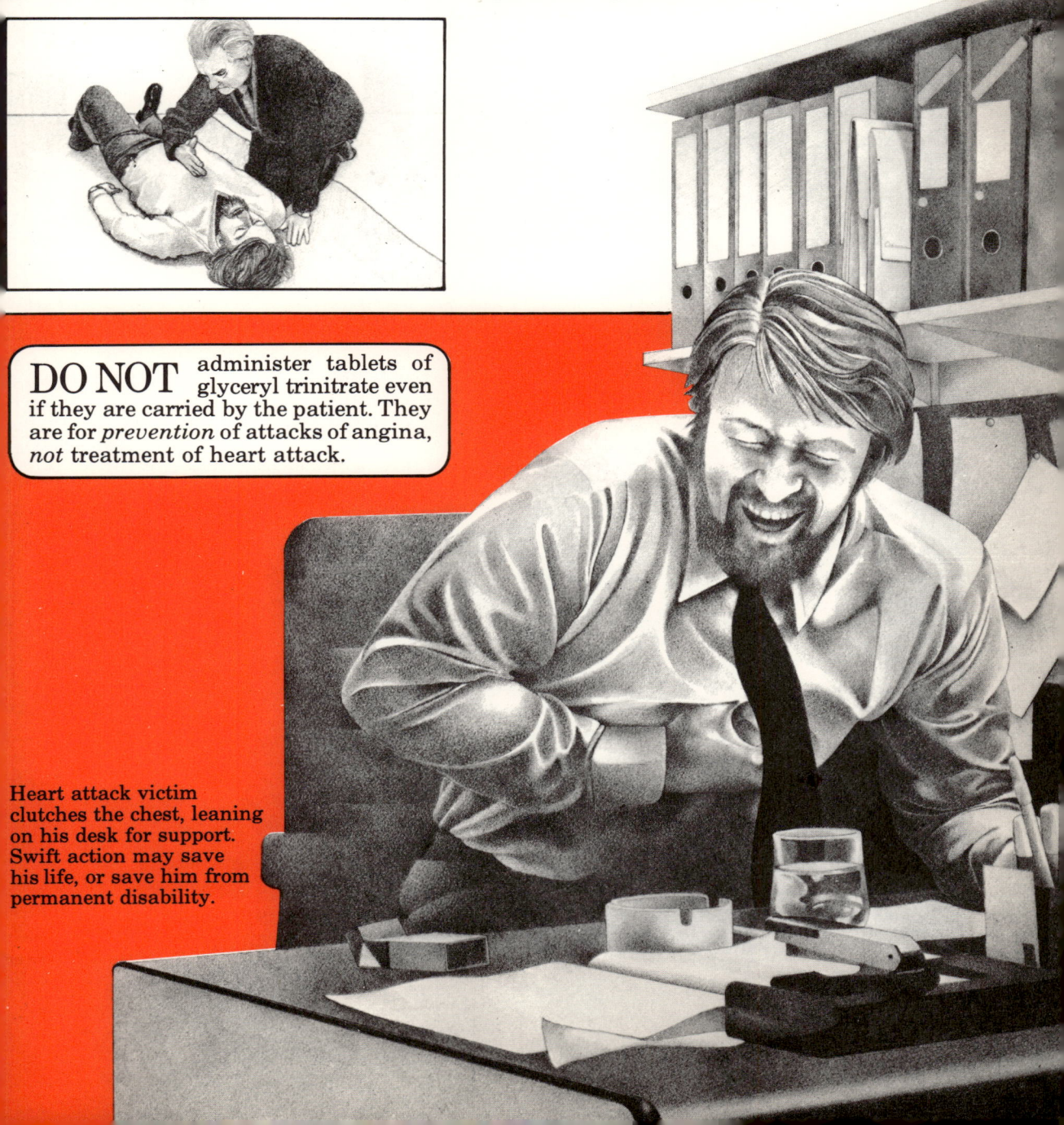

DO NOT administer tablets of glyceryl trinitrate even if they are carried by the patient. They are for *prevention* of attacks of angina, *not* treatment of heart attack.

Heart attack victim clutches the chest, leaning on his desk for support. Swift action may save his life, or save him from permanent disability.

Bleeding/Types of Wound

Rapid and profuse bleeding causes SHOCK (ACTION DETAILS **pp 90-91**) and if too much blood is lost, the result can be fatal. An adult in good health can lose up to a pint and a half of blood before the effect is serious but children and infants have far less blood and less than half a pint loss can be critical.

First aid priority is to stop the bleeding and get the casualty to a hospital immediately. A blood transfusion may mean the difference between life and death.

☎ *Summon an ambulance at once*

There are four main types of wound:
INCISED: A cut caused by a sharp instrument such as a knife or razor.
LACERATED: A torn, jagged wound caused by a sharp object such as a protruding nail.
CONTUSED: A bruising injury caused by a fall or a blow from a blunt instrument.
PUNCTURED: A small deep wound caused by a knife or by falling or treading on a nail.

Stopping severe bleeding

Blood will eventually clot of its own accord, but not while it is flowing profusely. If possible, raise the injured part of the body, but check first that there are no fractures or dislocations. Apply pressure to the wound, grasping the edges and forcing them together. Maintain pressure for about ten minutes to allow a clot to form. At the same time, try and get the casualty lying down with the head lowered. A dressing should be pressed onto the wound as soon as blood-flow eases. In an emergency, improvise: use a handkerchief, tie or scarf rolled into a pad. Arresting profuse bleeding is more important than worrying unduly about infection. When the flow has stopped, wipe away any *loose* dirt or foreign objects in the wound, using a clean swab. Finally, apply a clean dressing, pressing it firmly onto the wound, and bandage it firmly in place. If bleeding restarts, do not remove the dressing; add another on top of the first and bind in place. *Do not* attempt to move anything deeply embedded in a wound; this requires expert treatment and first aid should consist of applying a ring bandage (DETAILS **p 65**) and getting the casualty to a hospital as quickly as possible.

Keep talking to the casualty while you are attending to the injury. The sight of blood, and the scene of the accident, can be very frightening. *Constant reassurance is an important part of first aid.*

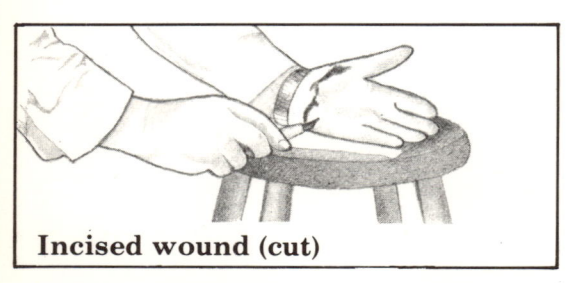

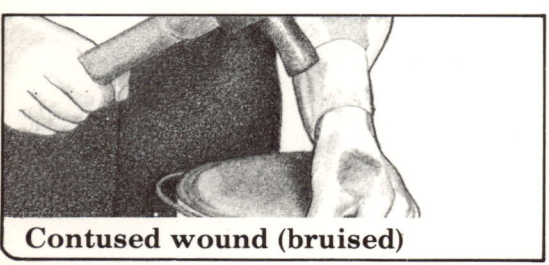

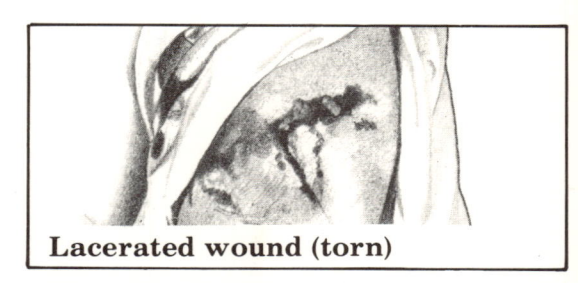

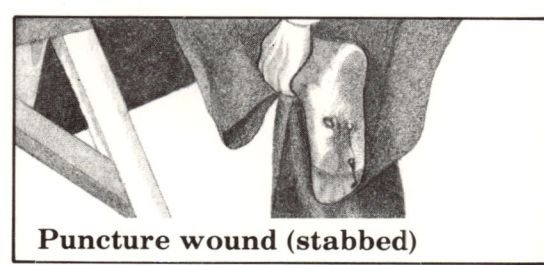

Incised wound (cut)

Lacerated wound (torn)

Contused wound (bruised)

Puncture wound (stabbed)

Internal bleeding

Internal bleeding around the ends of broken bones or within the body due to crushing injuries, can be just as deadly as visible bleeding. Signs include cold, clammy skin; rapid, feeble pulse; faintness or dizziness; fast labored breathing; sighing and complaints of feeling thirsty. There may be external signs such as bruising of the skin of the abdomen or bleeding from the nose or ears. If the chest is injured, frothy blood may be coughed up from the lungs. Keep the casualty warm and reassured and summon an ambulance urgently. Do not give the casualty any food or drink, but moisten his lips with water if he is distressed by feelings of thirst. If the chest or abdomen is injured, place a chair or small table over the casualty to keep the weight of coats or blankets off the body.

Treating slight bleeding

With less serious injuries, first wash your hands – keeping the wound temporarily covered with a clean handkerchief or towel – then wash the skin around the injury with soapy water or antiseptic. Wipe outward, away from the wound, and use each swab only once. Dry the wound and cover with a sterile dressing, making sure not to touch the sterile pad. Minor injuries should heal quickly but if any inflammation develops or if the wound appears to require stitching to avoid an unsightly scar, seek medical attention.

It is worth remembering that some antiseptics are harmful to open body tissue; but most antiseptic creams *can* be used on minor cuts and help inhibit infection. Used on dressings, they can help prevent sticking to the wounds.

The pressure points

Sometimes it proves impossible to stem severe bleeding by the normal method of applying direct pressure to the wound. In this emergency situation try to stop the flow by pushing on one of the pressure points between the wound site and the heart. Many pressure points are difficult to locate and use successfully without considerable experience but two are accessible to the first aider.

The BRACHIAL PRESSURE POINT is on the brachial artery which runs alongside the muscles on the inside of the upper arm. It should be compressed against the bone with the fingertips as illustrated. The FEMORAL PRESSURE POINT is located where the femoral artery runs into the leg at the center of the fold of the groin. The knee should be raised and the upper thigh grasped with both hands. With one thumb on top of the other press the artery against the pelvis.

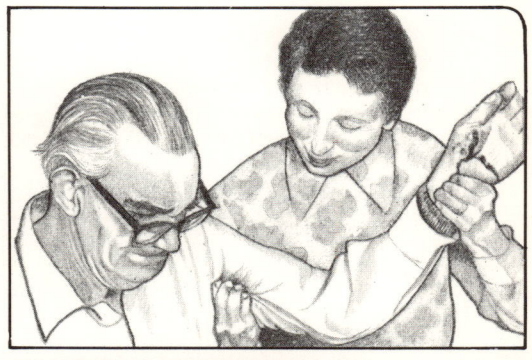

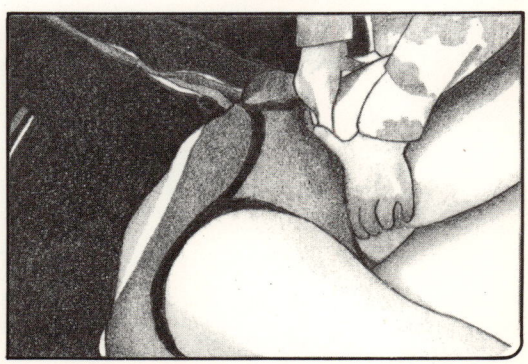

Bleeding/Arm and Hand

Upper arm - laceration

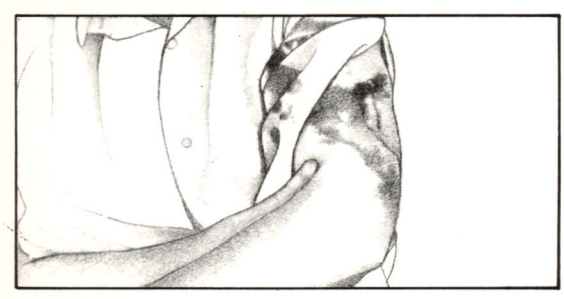

1 Clotting, encouraged by application of pressure, will arrest the flow of blood.

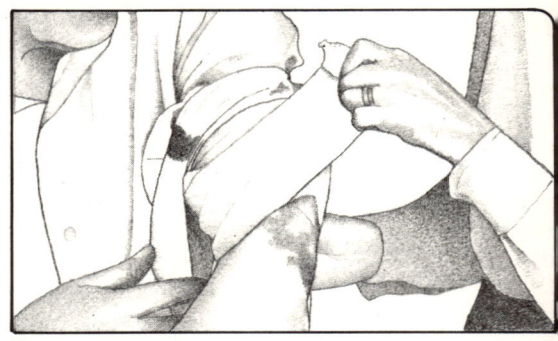

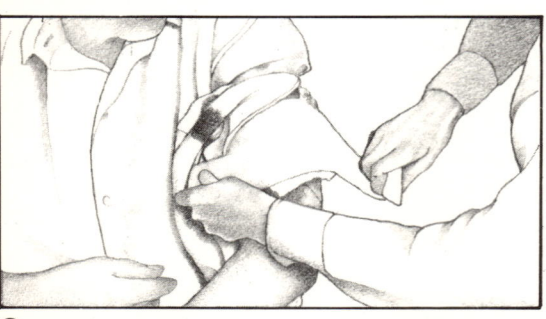

2 If no foreign matter is embedded in the wound, apply a large dressing pad.

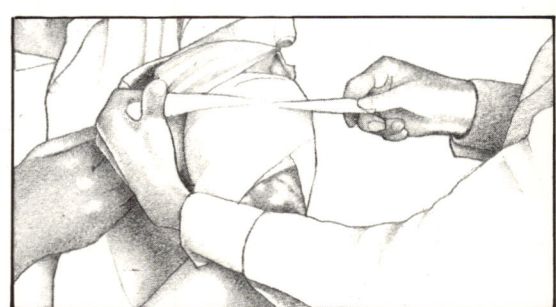

3 Bandage firmly to maintain pressure but do not impede circulation.

4 Tie off the bandage with a square knot well clear of the site of the injury.

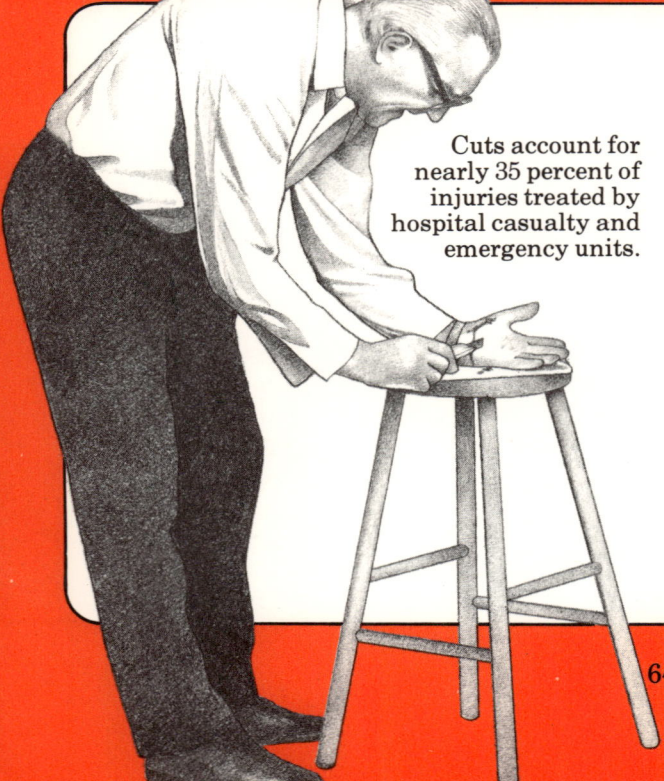

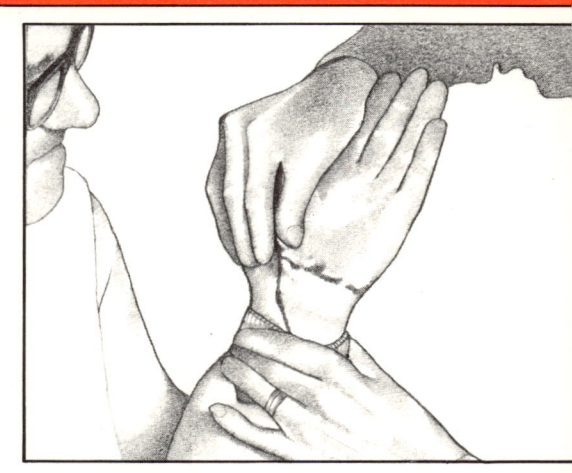

Cuts account for nearly 35 percent of injuries treated by hospital casualty and emergency units.

Hand injury - incised wound

1 Keep the injured hand as high as possible to reduced blood flow. Pinch the sides of the wound firmly together to promote clotting.

Ring bandage

If a piece of metal, wood or glass is deeply embedded in the wound, *on no account try to pull it out.* You will make the injury worse and almost certainly initiate renewed bleeding. Gently swab dirt away from the wound, taking care not to press on the injury. Make a ring-bandage as illustrated and place this over the wound. Bandage over the pad.

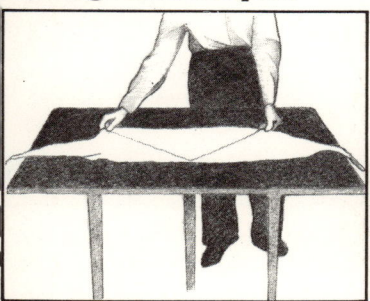

1 Take a triangular bandage and fold lengthways.

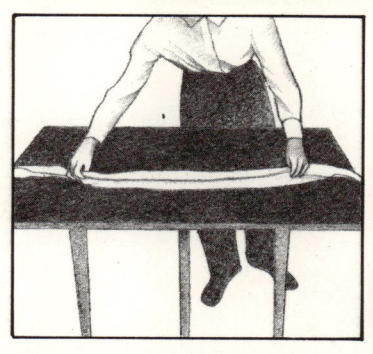

2 Fold the bandage down to a band 2 inches wide.

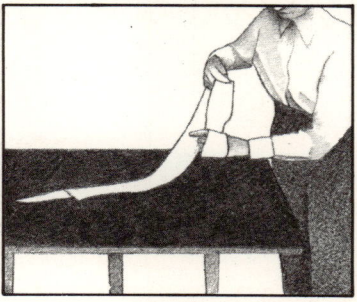

3 Loop the bandage round the hand to make a ring.

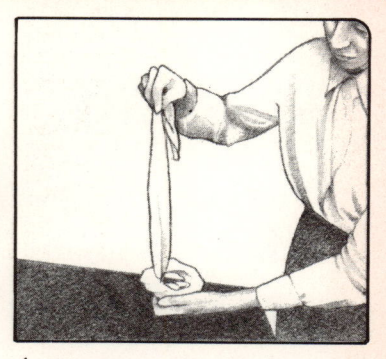

4 Bind the remaining bandage tightly around the loop.

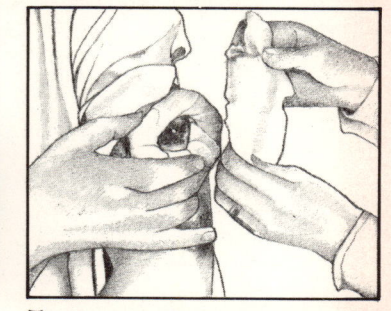

5 Place the ring over the wound: bandage in place.

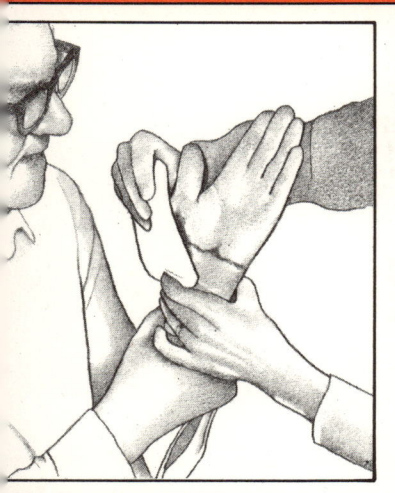

As soon as the flow of blood eases, or is reduced to minor seepage, press a clean dressing firmly onto the wound.

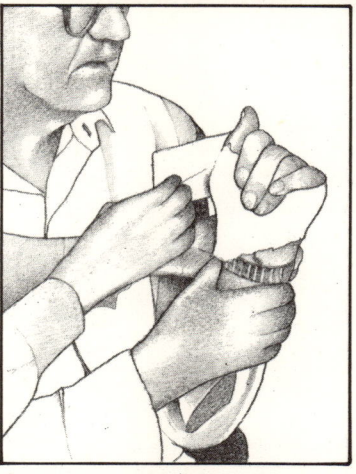

3 Bandage the dressing in place firmly enough to maintain pressure but do not impede circulation.

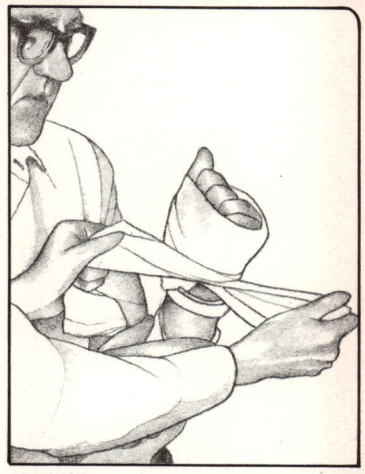

4 Finish off with several turns round the hand. Take the casualty to a hospital, keeping the hand raised.

Bleeding/Foot, Knee and Elbow

Foot - puncture wound

Although puncture wounds seldom bleed heavily they require medical attention immediately due to the risk of infection and, if deep, possible internal bleeding. Clean the wound and apply a dry dressing. Bandage with a triangular bandage (**this page**) or with a figure-eight (**see pp 84-5**) and take the casualty to hospital.

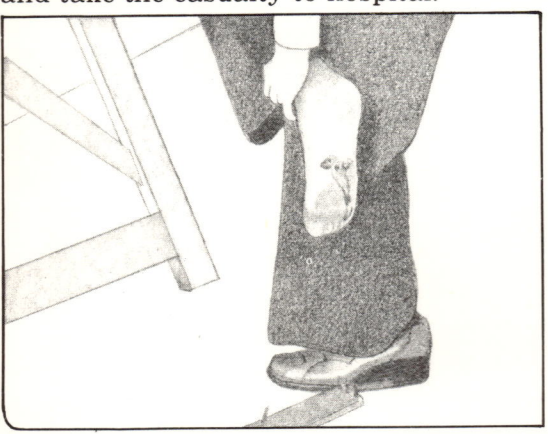

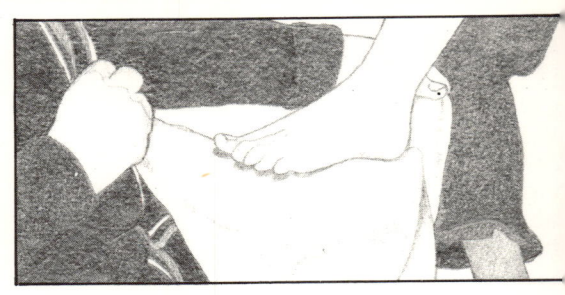

1 Place the foot on the bandage with the he about 4 in. from the centre of the long edg

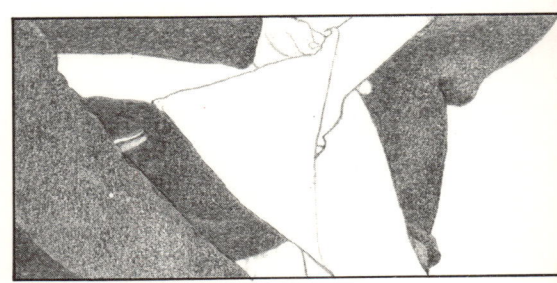

2 Lift the front corner of the bandage over the foot and ask the casualty to hold

Knee - triangular bandage

Although any damage to the joint itself should be supported by padding and an elasticized bandage (**See SPRAIN, ACTION DETAILS pp 84-5**), cuts and grazes on the knee are most easily bandaged using a triangular bandage. The wound should first be cleaned with soapy water or mild antiseptic solution. If the wound is dirty or becomes inflamed, seek medical attention.

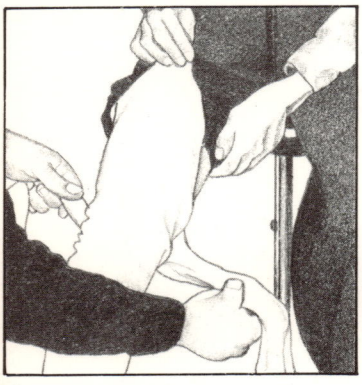

1 Place a dry dressing over the injury and cover with the bandage, crossing the long ends below the knee.

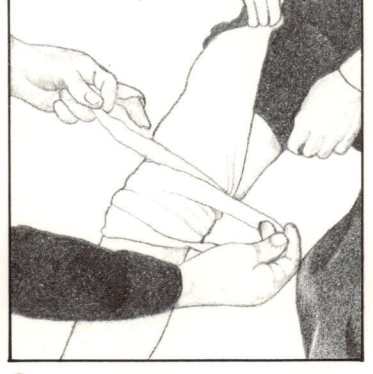

2 The long ends of the bandage are taken behind the knee and up onto the thigh just above the knee.

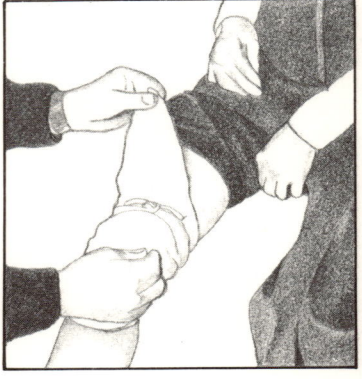

3 Tie off with a square knot; take the protruding corner of the bandage down and pin securely over the knot.

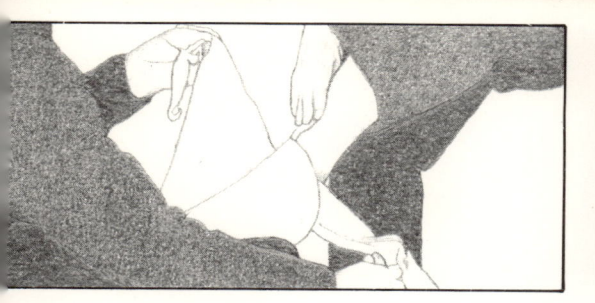

Take one side of the bandage across the top of the foot and round the back of the heel.

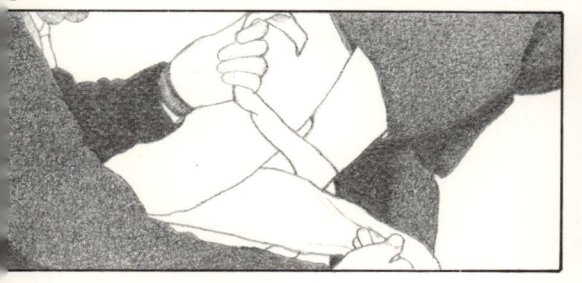

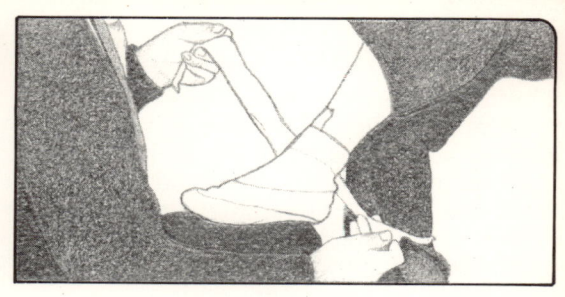

5 Bring both ends of the bandage to the front and tie firmly with a square knot.

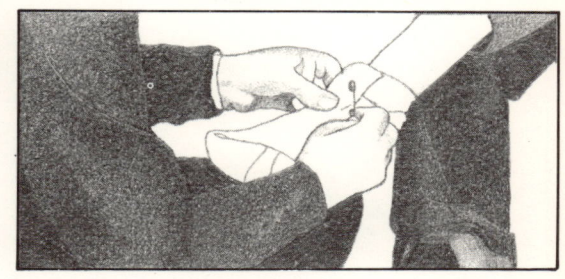

Changing hands if more convenient, repeat with the other side of the bandage.

6 Finish by turning down the protruding corner and pinning it over the knot.

Elbow - gauze bandage

Minor injuries at or near the elbow are common and include burns from contact with hot pipes or pans, grazes suffered playing football and other games, or deep scratches caused by protruding nails or door catches. The injury should be carefully cleaned with an antiseptic solution and covered with a dry dressing before being bandaged. If any injury fails to heal quickly, seek medical attention.

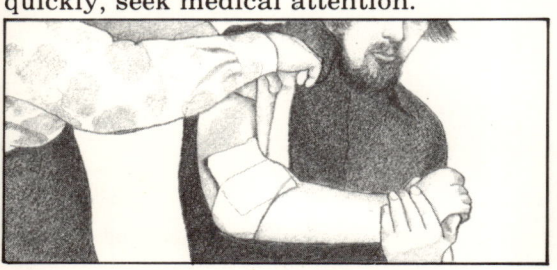

1 Anchor the bandage by taking two turns round the arm close to the elbow.

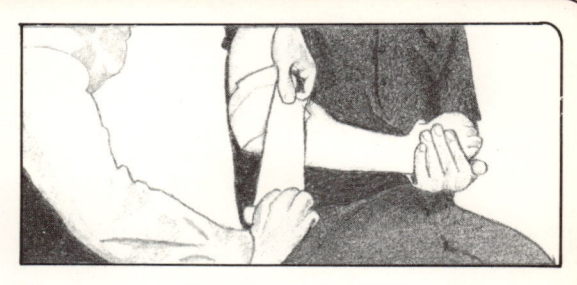

2 Make two or three turns alternately above and below the angle of the elbow.

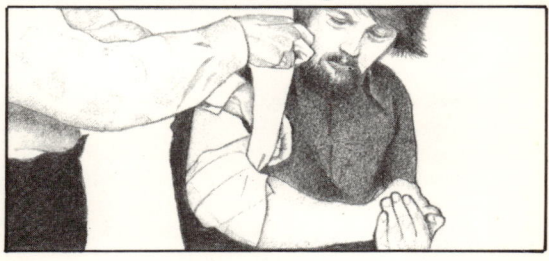

3 A more comfortable result is achieved by twisting the bandage between turns.

Bleeding/Finger

Finger – gauze bandage

The fingers are naturally very vulnerable to cuts but even the most minor injury should be immediately – and carefully – cleaned and dressed to avoid complications due to infection. This is particularly important if the injury is suffered while gardening or handling dirty materials in the garage or workshop.

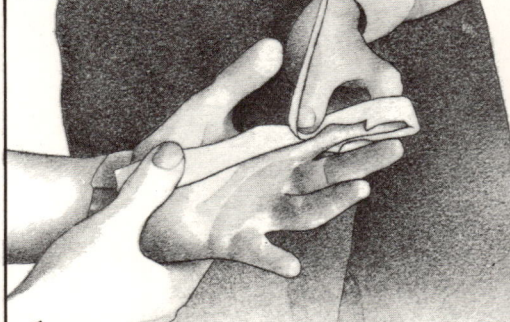

Small cuts may be simply covered with an adhesive plaster dressing but deeper or more extensive injuries should be bandaged. Tubular finger-bandages are by far the most convenient, and secure, but are not always readily available. The illustrations, right, demonstrate the correct method using a standard roll of 1-inch-wide gauze bandage.

1 With the casualty's help, lay the bandage along the finger, down the back, and return to the front.

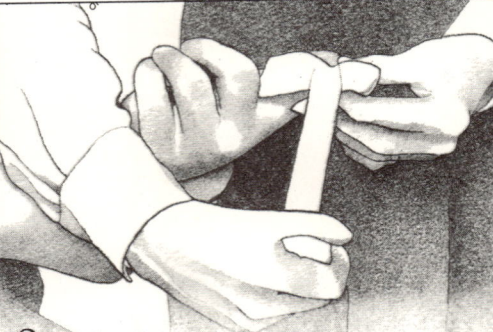

2 Take the bandage back to the tip of the finger, tuck in the corners and start bandaging round the finger.

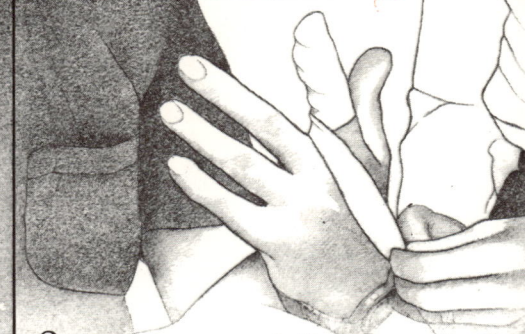

3 Bandage round the finger to the base, overlapping each turn by about two-thirds the width of the bandage.

Head 68/69

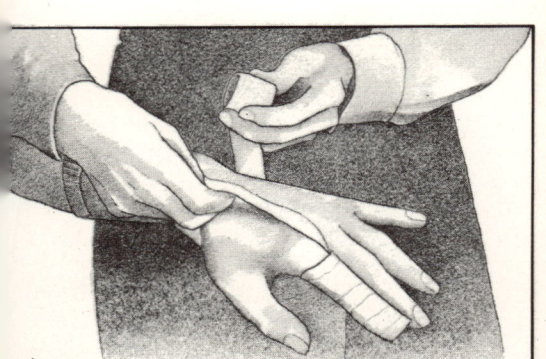

4 Lay the bandage along the back of the hand, take a turn round the wrist and pass beneath the fixed part.

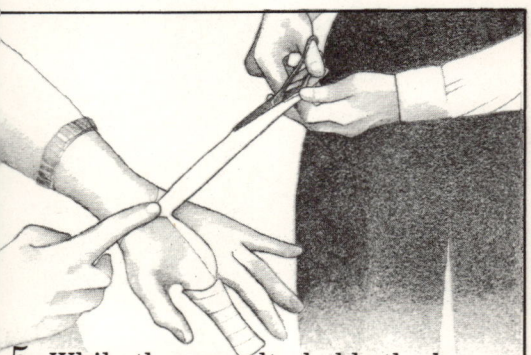

5 While the casualty holds the bandage in place, trim off the excess and split the loose end along its length.

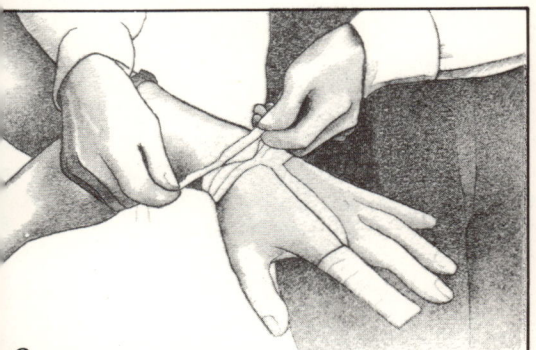

6 Tie the two strands to prevent further splitting, then tie them firmly around the wrist using a square knot.

Head injury

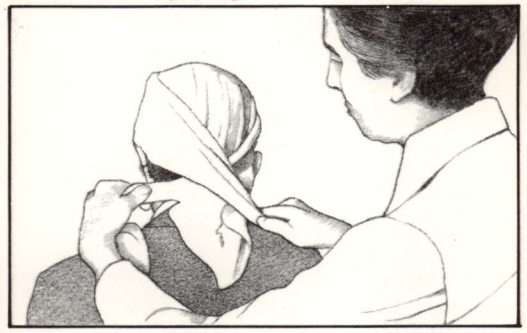

1 Place a dressing pad over the injury and cover with the triangular bandage, crossing the long ends behind the head.

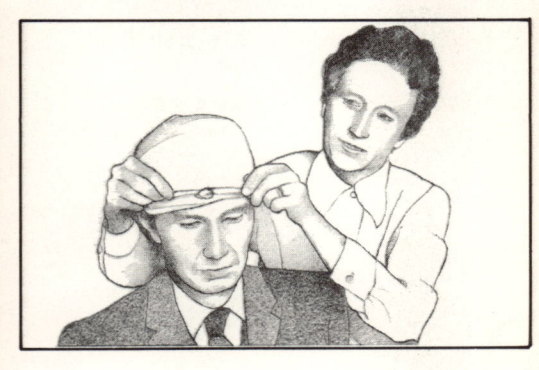

2 Take the ends around to the front and tie with a square knot over the forehead. Tuck in the loose ends.

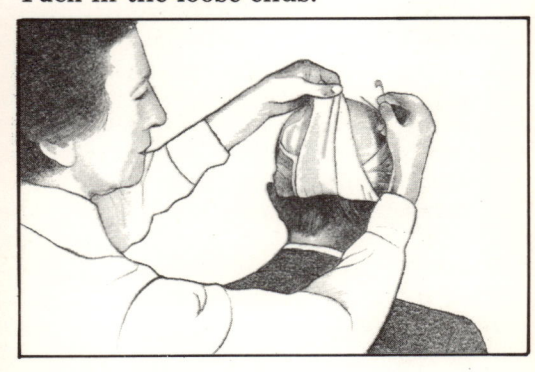

3 Tidy up the back by folding up the protruding corner of the bandage and pinning it at the back of the head.

Loss of Consciousness

There are many different causes of loss of consciousness – asphyxia, head injury, poisoning, shock, heart attack, epilepsy, stroke and diabetic crisis among them – but the primary task of first aid is not to find the reason but to take prompt emergency action to keep the victim alive until he can receive expert attention.

There are two priorities

To prevent and relieve any obstruction to the patient's breathing and to

☎ *Summon a doctor or ambulance as quickly as possible.*

The greatest danger is that of suffocation. The most common cause is the casualty's limp tongue falling back and blocking the windpipe, but blood, vomit, saliva, even loose teeth, can cause an obstruction. Always clear the mouth out thoroughly with your fingers or with a handkerchief.

IF THE CASUALTY IS NOT BREATHING you must begin **ARTIFICIAL RESPIRATION** immediately (ACTION DETAILS **pp 52-7**).

IF HE IS BREATHING keep his head well down and tilted back, and pull the jaw forward to move the tongue clear of the windpipe. Turn the head to one side to allow any fluids to drain from the mouth.

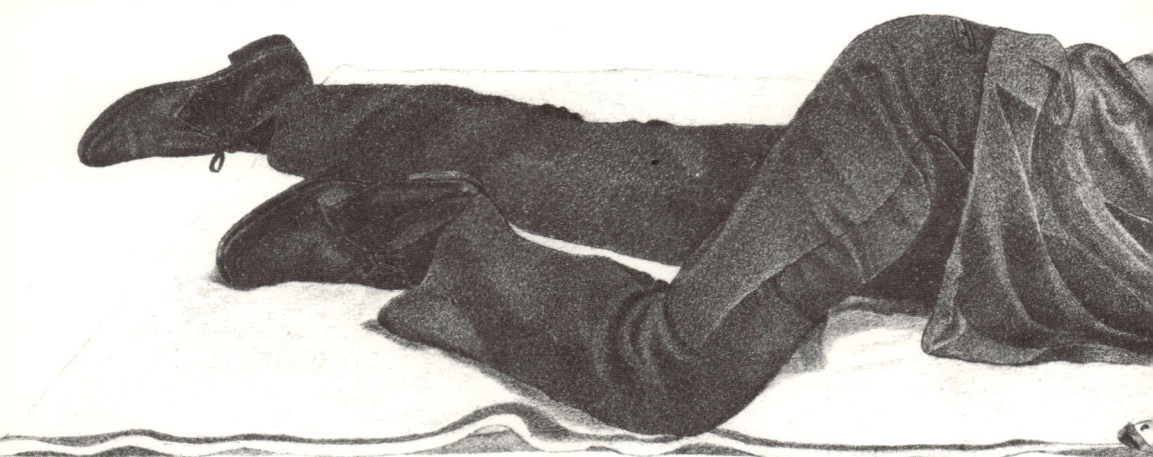

The recovery position

Ideally you should get the casualty into the recovery position as soon as possible but first check carefully to ensure that there are no major fractures. Feel along the limbs, pelvis and spine for swelling or deformities which may indicate broken bones or internal injury. *If serious injury is suspected do not move the casualty*, but stay by his head keeping the breathing passages clear and unobstructed.

The recovery position allows the unconscious person to breathe more easily and prevents fluids like saliva or vomit from collecting in the throat. If fluids are breathed into the lungs they can cause serious complications - including severe, and possibly fatal, pneumonia.

To place the casualty in the recovery position, kneel beside him and position his arms close to his sides. Cross the far leg over the nearer one; cradle the face with one hand and with the other pull the hip up and over toward you.

Now position the leg and arm nearer to you in the position illustrated above. These limbs act as props, preventing the casualty from rolling onto his face. Finally, make sure that the face is tilted slightly downward (again for drainage) and the head bent back with the chin pulled forward to keep the airways clear. Do not use a pillow. If the patient was in bed remove the pillows and raise the foot of the bed. Loosen any restricting clothing.

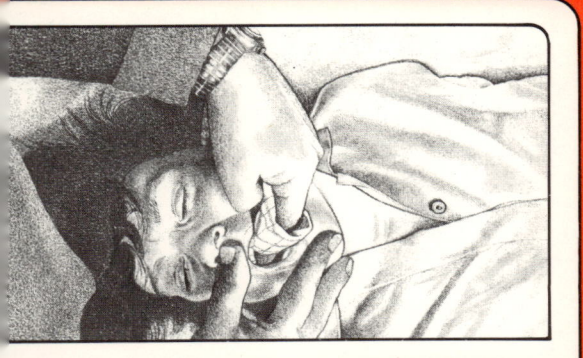

DO NOT give the casualty any food or drink or leave him unattended, but moisten his lips when he recovers.

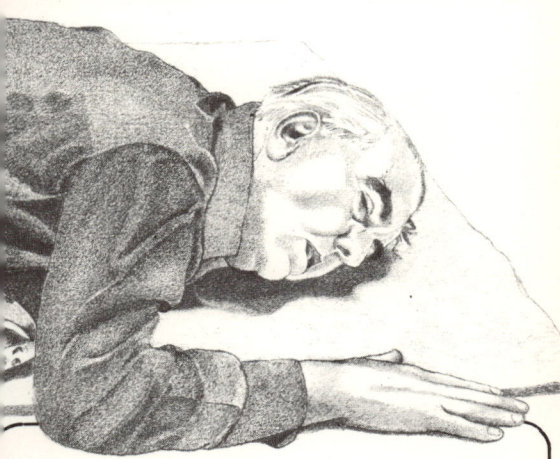

CONCUSSION, caused by a sudden shaking of the brain inside the skull, may cause unconsciousness for only a few seconds and the casualty may then feel alright. But anyone who has been knocked out – even momentarily – should be seen by a doctor and anyone who has difficulty with speech or co-ordination should go to a hospital.

While waiting for expert help you can check for, and treat, BLEEDING (ACTION DETAILS **pp 62-9**); BROKEN BONES (ACTION DETAILS **72-83**), and keep the casualty warm with a blanket or coat. On regaining consciousness he should be treated for SHOCK (DETAILS **pp90-91**).

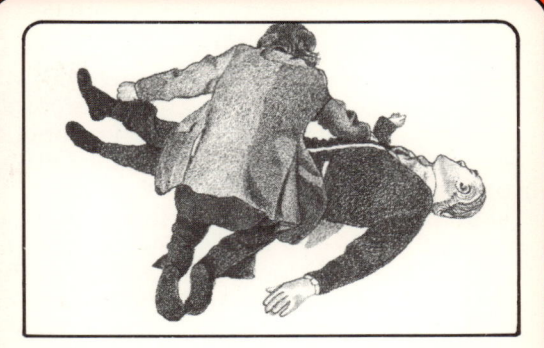

To move a casualty into the recovery position, tuck his arms in close to his sides and pull the far leg toward you.

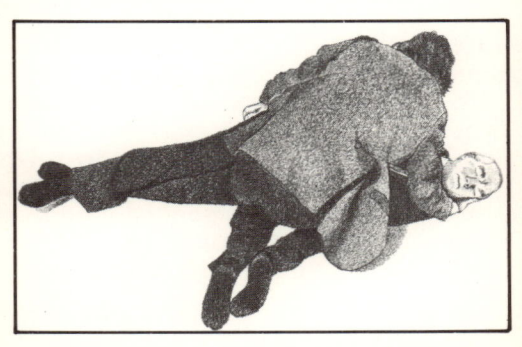

Cradling the face with your right hand pull the hip up and over. A sharp pull will turn even a heavy casualty.

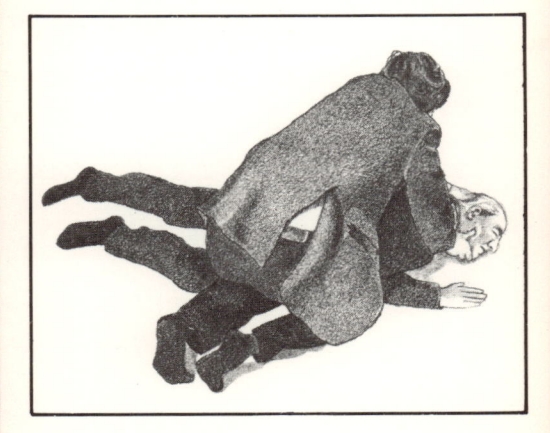

Arrange the arms and legs as shown to support the body and ease breathing; the head should be tilted well back.

Broken Bones

A bone may break either directly at the spot where the blow was received or at a point some distance away from the point of contact. A fracture of the collarbone, for example, may result from a fall onto the outstretched hand, while a fracture of the skull may be caused by a blow to the lower jaw or by a heavy jarring fall onto the feet or the base of the spine. Occasionally a fracture may be caused by a sudden and violent contraction of the muscles attached to the bone, as in a violent electric shock. *If in doubt, treat any very painful injury as a possible fracture.*

The majority of fractures fall into two main categories: COMPOUND, or OPEN, fractures where the bone penetrates the skin and the wound is thus open to infection, and SIMPLE, or CLOSED, fractures where the bone is not exposed. The latter may, however, be complicated by internal bleeding or by injury to internal organs. A third type, more commonly found in children, is the GREENSTICK fracture which involves partial breaking of the bone.

Action details

First priority should be to deal with BREATHING STOPPAGE (ACTION DETAILS **pp 52-7**), BLEEDING (**pp 62-9**) and SHOCK (**pp 90-91**). Then: immobilize the injured part, moving the casualty as little as possible; keep the casualty calm and reassured, and . . .

☎ *Telephone for an ambulance.*

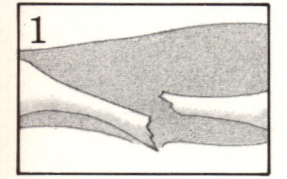

1 Compound fracture; bone exposed.

2 Simple fracture, skin not broken.

3 Greenstick type

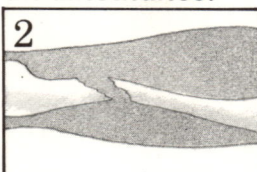

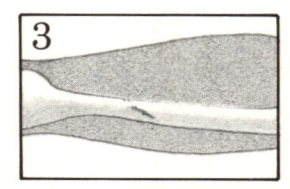

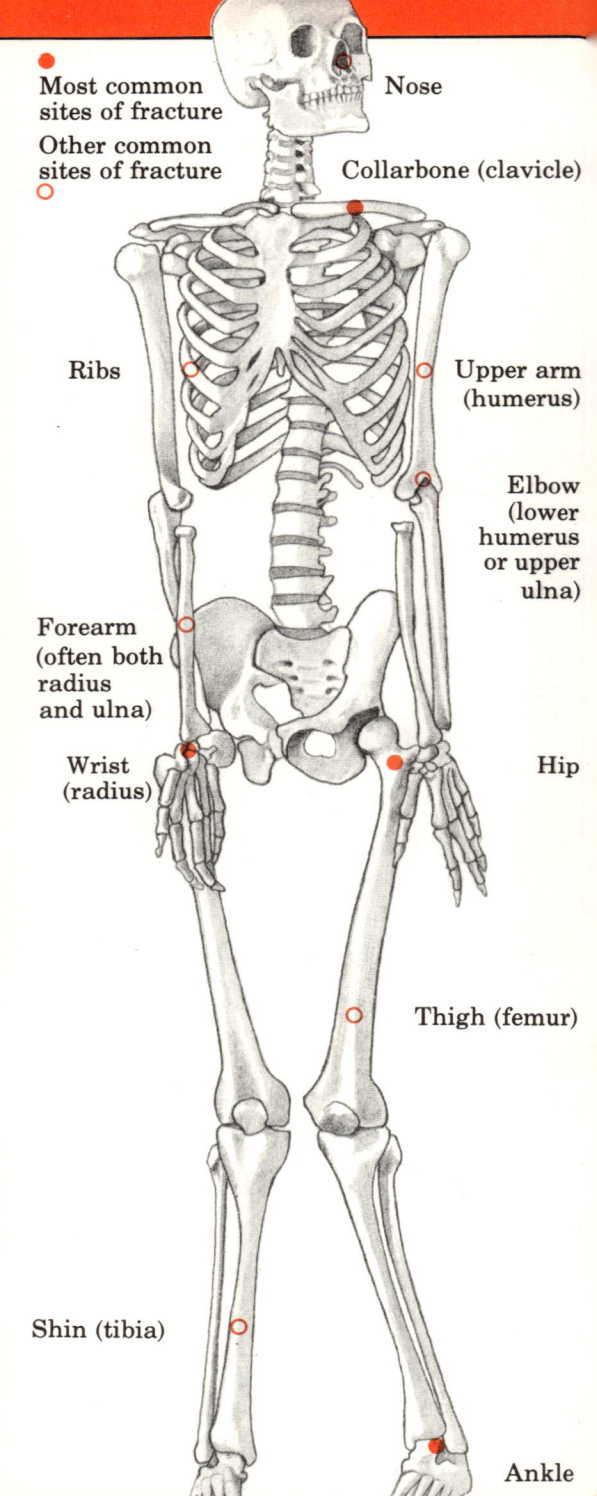

- ● Most common sites of fracture
- ○ Other common sites of fracture

- Nose
- Collarbone (clavicle)
- Ribs
- Upper arm (humerus)
- Elbow (lower humerus or upper ulna)
- Forearm (often both radius and ulna)
- Wrist (radius)
- Hip
- Thigh (femur)
- Shin (tibia)
- Ankle

Arm, Elbow and Hand 72/73

Upper arm and forearm

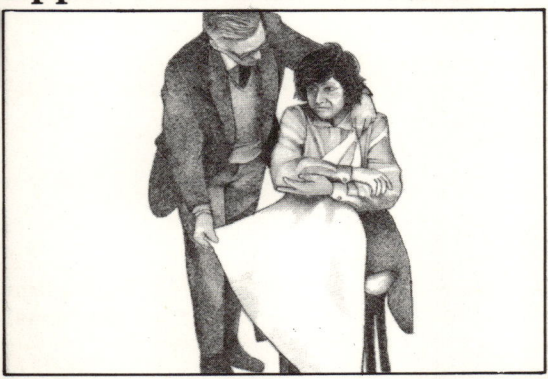

1 While the casualty supports the injured arm, gently draw a triangular bandage up to the shoulder between the arm and body.

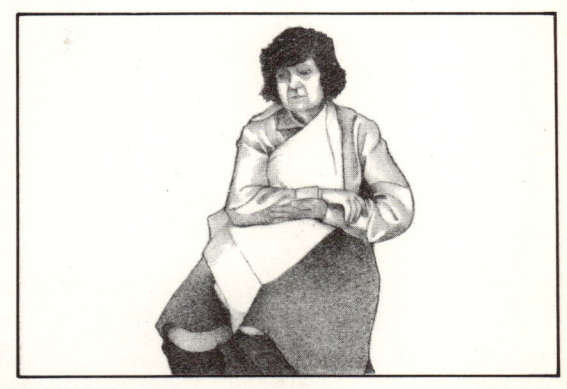

2 Place a soft pad – cotton, handkerchief, folded scarf or pullover – between the injured arm and the casualty's body.

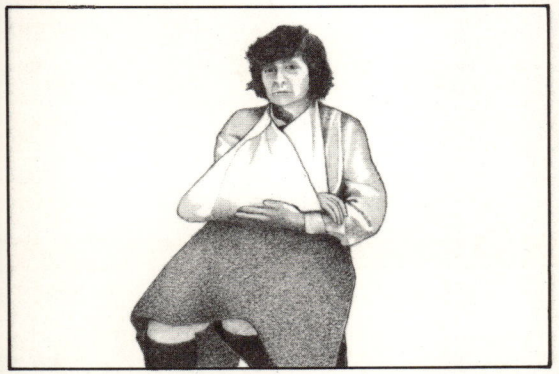

3 Raise the other half of the bandage and secure with a square knot. The third corner is taken behind the elbow and pinned.

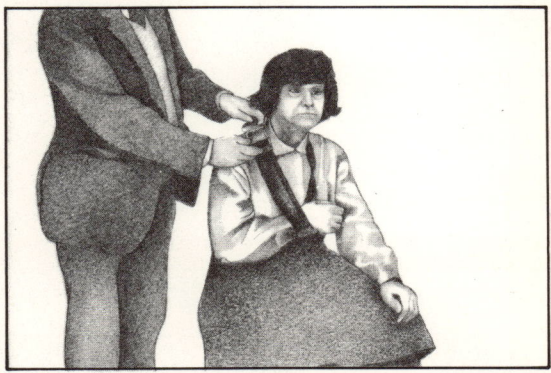

4 If a triangular bandage is not available, a temporary sling can be made from a belt, necktie or woman's stocking.

Elbow

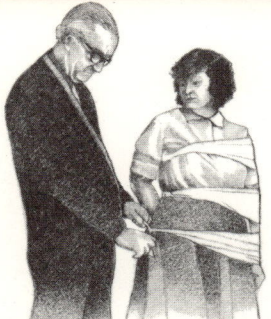

If a broken elbow is bent, support it in a sling as above. If straight, immobilize at the side with three broad bandages.

Hand

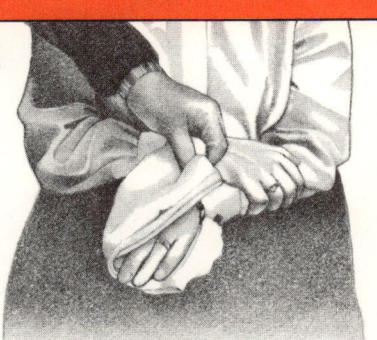

Gently bend the elbow and protect the injured hand in a fold of soft padding. The arm should then be put in a sling.

Broken Bones/Lower Leg and Thigh

Symptoms of a break will be severe pain and difficulty in moving the limb. The leg may also look unnatural due to swelling or to being displaced from its normal position. Comparing the two limbs will often help in deciding if a fracture has occurred, but *if in doubt treat any leg injury as a fracture* until expert advice is available.

Fractures of the leg bones, and particularly of the thigh, are nearly always accompanied by SHOCK (ACTION DETAILS **pp 90-91**). Casualties must be moved as little as possible – and then only with the use of a stretcher. In an emergency a door or section of fencing, or even a short ladder, may be used.

Bandages should be tied firmly but not so tight that they impede circulation. They should be checked every 15 minutes to make sure that swelling has not made them too tight. Knots should always be tied on the casualty's uninjured side or, where splints are used, over the splint.

☎ *Telephone for an ambulance as quickly as possible.*

Broken leg – easy journey

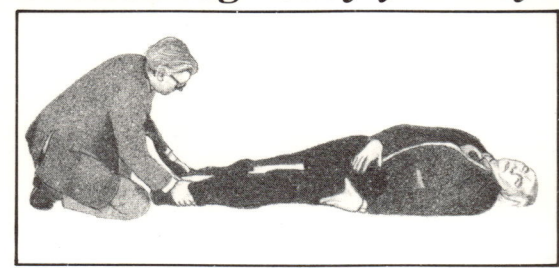

1 Gently bring the legs into line. Place pads between the thighs, knees and ankles.

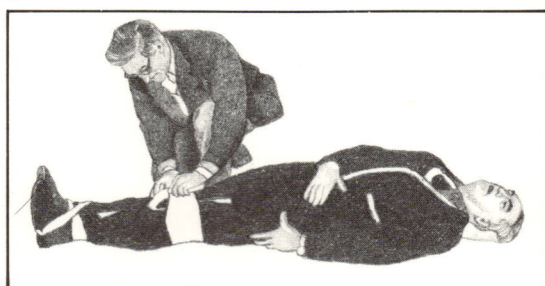

2 Bind the feet and ankles with a figure-eight, and the knees with a broad band.

Broken leg – using splints

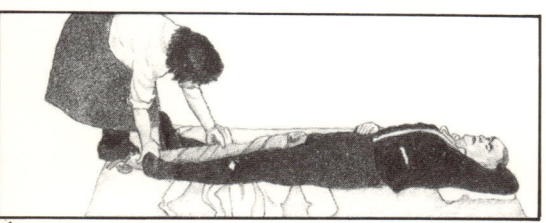

1 A well-padded splint should be placed between the legs from crotch to heel.

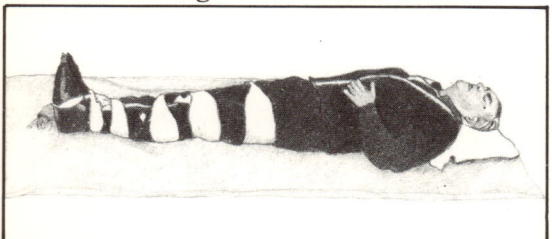

2 Five bandages should be tied round the splinted legs as shown in the upper panel.

Fractured thigh

The thigh bone is the largest bone in the body and can only be broken by a very violent blow. Consequently any fracture of the thigh will be accompanied by SHOCK (ACTION DETAILS **pp 90-91**) and quite possibly by other fractures or internal injuries depending on the circumstances. If fracture of the thigh is suspected, the casualty must be moved as little as possible, and *only by stretcher*.

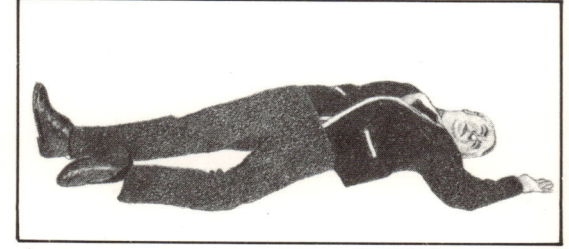

1 Fracture of the thigh may be revealed by the leg and foot being turned outward.

Broken leg – more difficult journey

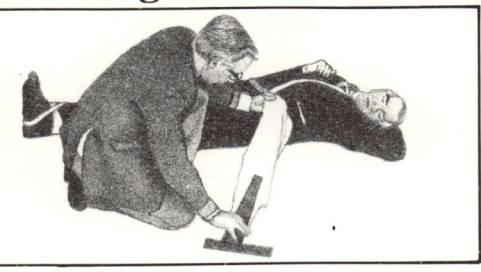

1. The additional bandages needed may be passed under the body using a stick.

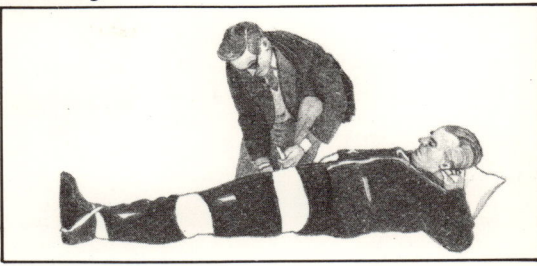

2. Tie a broad bandage round the upper thighs and another at mid-thigh level.

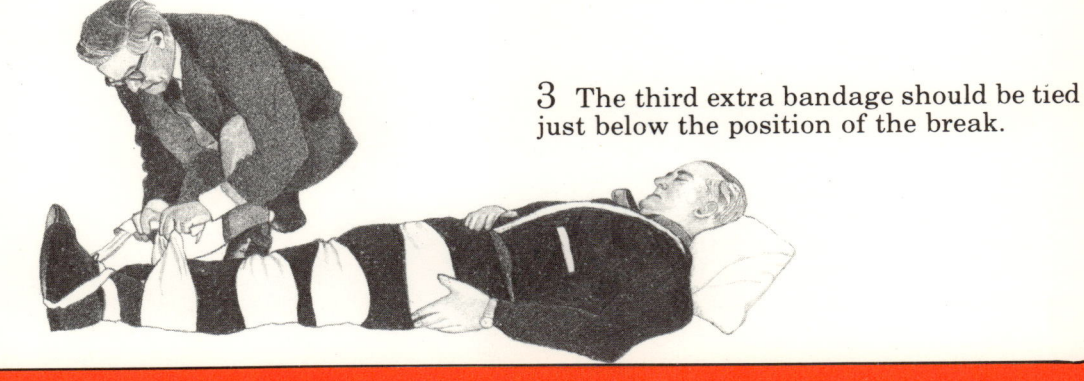

3. The third extra bandage should be tied just below the position of the break.

2. If straightening the leg causes excessive pain, stop and pad the leg where it is.

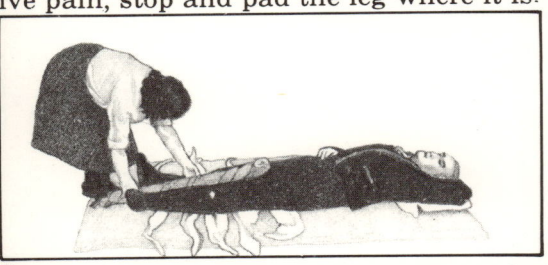

3. Place a well-padded splint between the legs from crotch to just past the heel.

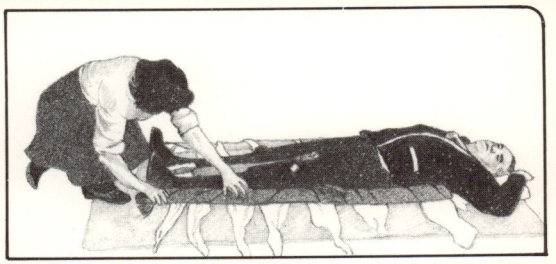

4. Place a long padded splint along the body from the armpit to the heel.

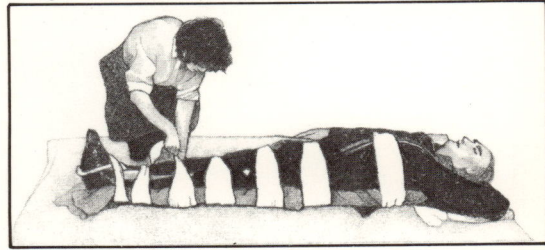

5. Bandage as in the upper panel, with two additional bandages round hips and chest.

Broken Bones/Knee

The kneecap can be broken by a direct blow or fall onto it or, more rarely, it may be broken by violent contraction of the powerful muscles attached to it from the front of the thigh. The casualty should lie down with head and shoulders supported and the injured leg raised.

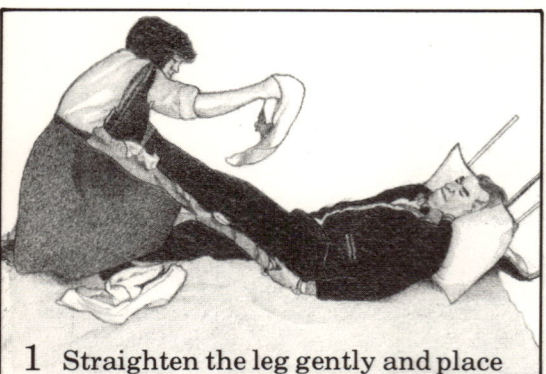

1 Straighten the leg gently and place a well-padded splint along the back of the leg from the buttock to the heel.

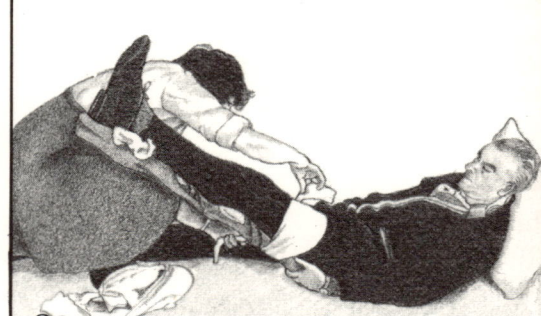

2 Supporting the injured leg on your thigh, place pads between the splint and leg behind the knee and ankle.

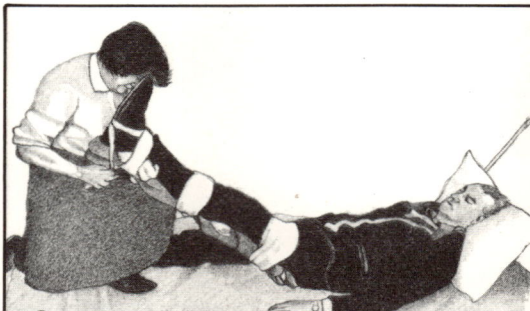

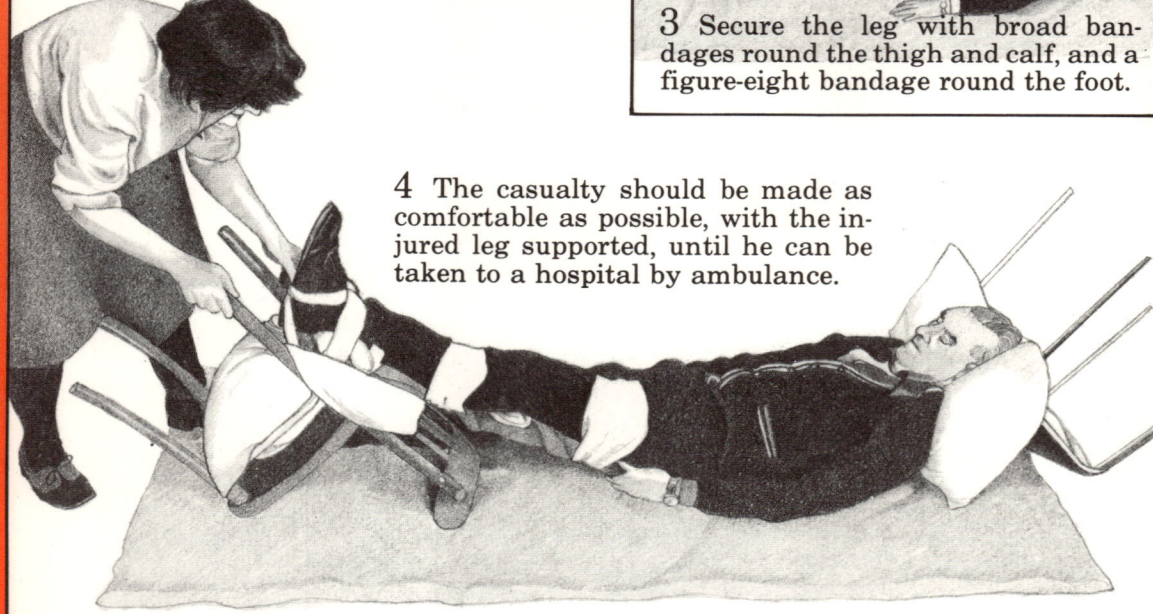

3 Secure the leg with broad bandages round the thigh and calf, and a figure-eight bandage round the foot.

4 The casualty should be made as comfortable as possible, with the injured leg supported, until he can be taken to a hospital by ambulance.

Foot

The majority of injuries to the bones of the foot are caused either by dropping a heavy weight onto the foot or by a heavy vehicle running over it.

Action details

The first emergency action should be to remove the shoe and the sock or stocking, as gently as possible, before the foot swells. If necessary the shoe should be cut away. The casualty should be made as comfortable as possible with the injured leg raised and supported, until he can be taken to a hospital for expert treatment.

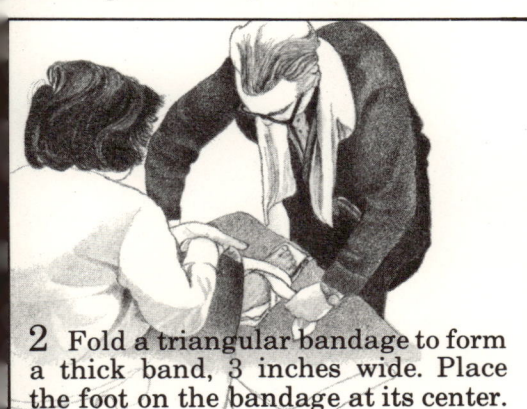

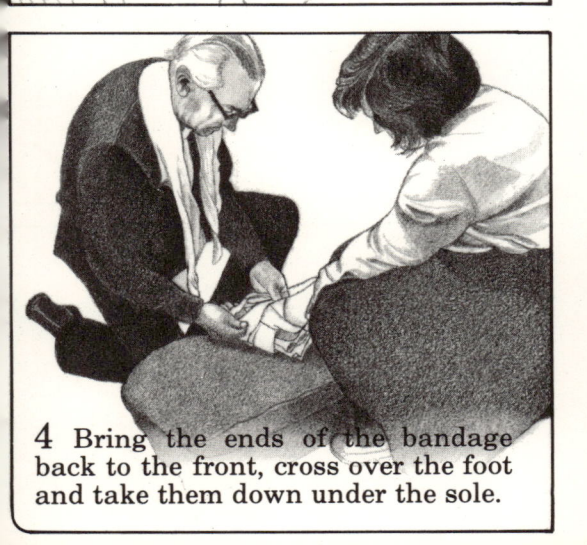

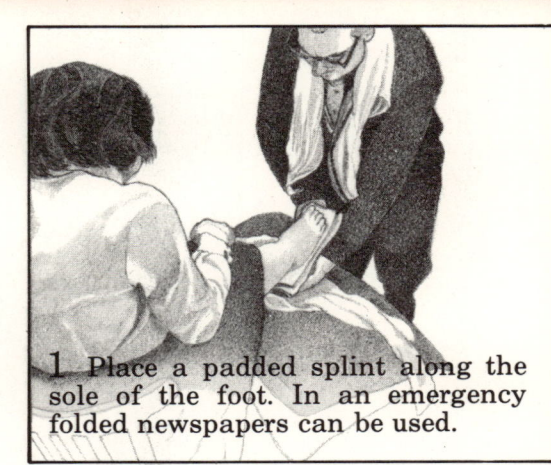

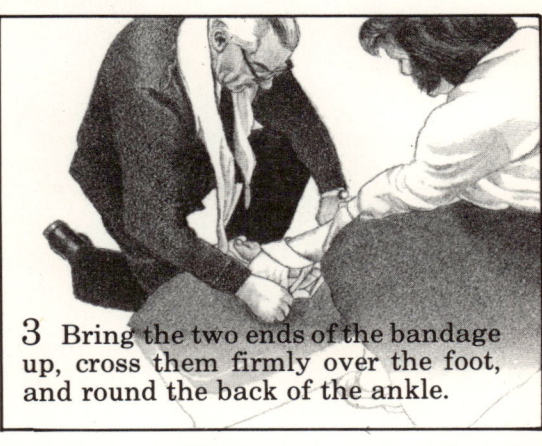

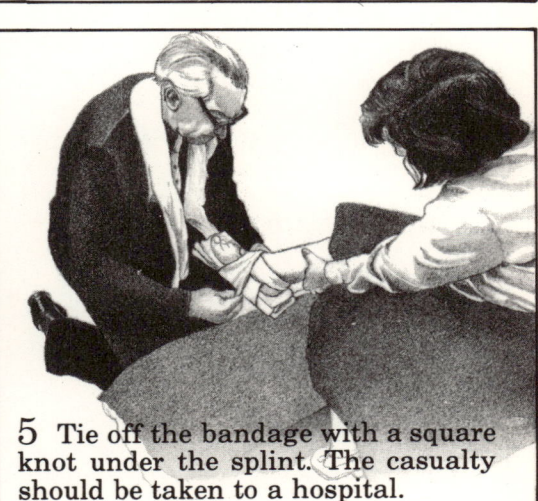

1 Place a padded splint along the sole of the foot. In an emergency folded newspapers can be used.

2 Fold a triangular bandage to form a thick band, 3 inches wide. Place the foot on the bandage at its center.

3 Bring the two ends of the bandage up, cross them firmly over the foot, and round the back of the ankle.

4 Bring the ends of the bandage back to the front, cross over the foot and take them down under the sole.

5 Tie off the bandage with a square knot under the splint. The casualty should be taken to a hospital.

Broken Bones/Spine

Signs and symptoms
The casualty will complain of severe pain in the back or neck, and possibly of a loss of feeling and control in the limbs. He must be handled with extreme care to avoid damage to the nerves in the spine.

☎ *Summon an ambulance at once*

Action details
Deal first with BREATHING STOPPAGES (see pp 52-7) and BLEEDING (pp 62-9).

If help can be summoned quickly, *do not move the casualty. Warn him to lie still.* Only if help is not available should you attempt to move him and for this you will

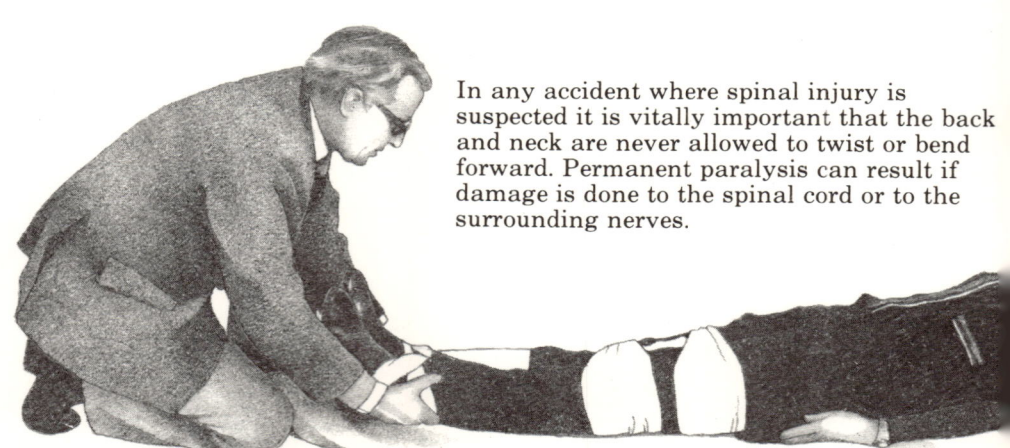

In any accident where spinal injury is suspected it is vitally important that the back and neck are never allowed to twist or bend forward. Permanent paralysis can result if damage is done to the spinal cord or to the surrounding nerves.

Lifting onto a stretcher
Any casualty suffering injury to the legs, pelvis or spine should be moved only by stretcher, using the following sequence.

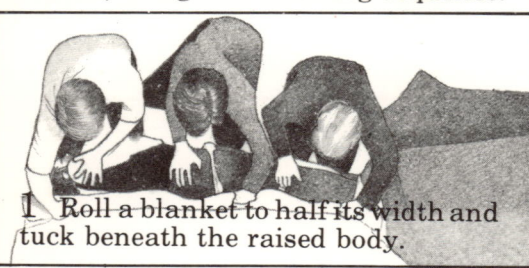

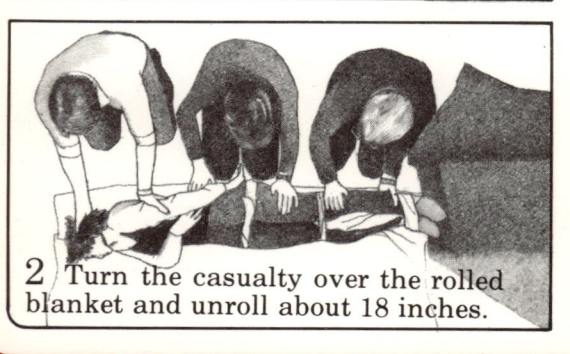

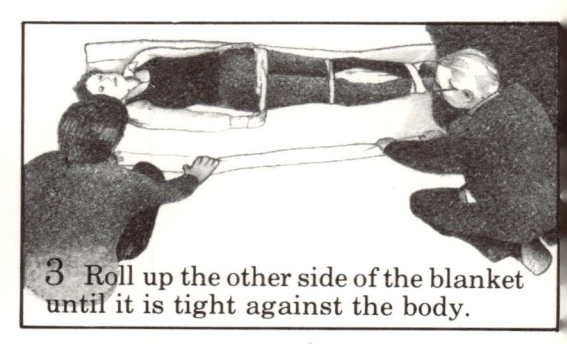

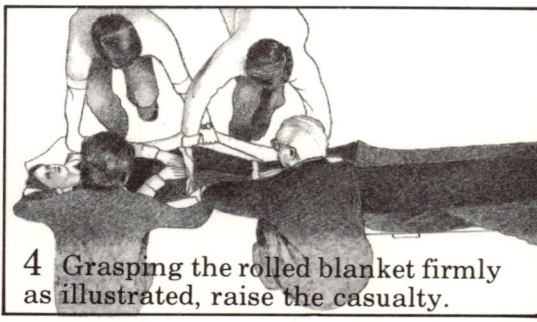

1 Roll a blanket to half its width and tuck beneath the raised body.

2 Turn the casualty over the rolled blanket and unroll about 18 inches.

3 Roll up the other side of the blanket until it is tight against the body.

4 Grasping the rolled blanket firmly as illustrated, raise the casualty.

Pelvis 78/79

...ed at least four people. At all times, one ...rson at the head and one at the feet ...ould keep the body in tension and *rigidly* ... *line*. Place pads between the thighs, ...ees and ankles; bind the feet with a ...gure-eight bandage and the knees with a ...oad band. The casualty may then be ...aced on a stretcher as illustrated below.

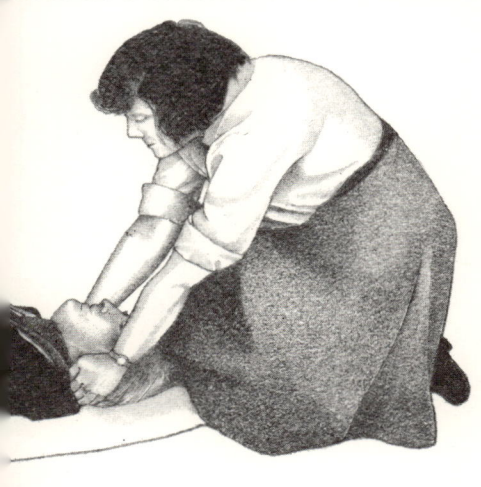

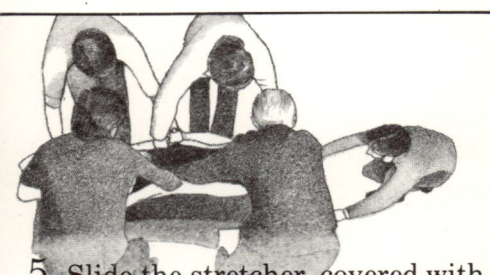

5 Slide the stretcher, covered with a blanket, underneath the casualty.

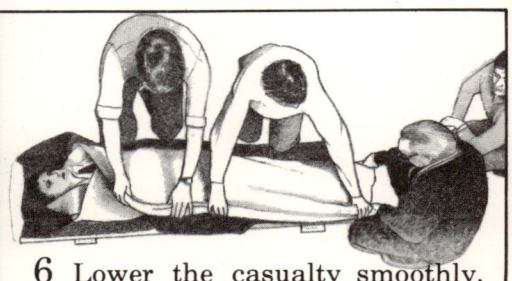

6 Lower the casualty smoothly, wrap the blanket tightly around.

Fracture of the pelvis may be complicated by injury to the internal organs, in particular the bladder and urinary passages. The casualty may feel that he wishes to pass water but should be warned to resist the urge as this may only worsen the injury.

The casualty will be unable to stand and should be allowed to lie on his back in the most comfortable position while help is summoned. If expert help will take long to arrive, and it is necessary to take the casualty to a hospital, he should be firmly bandaged as illustrated and moved by stretcher.

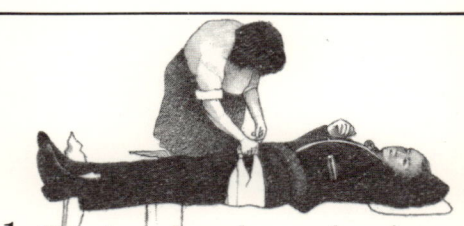

1 Tie two broad, overlapping bandages round the hips, tying off over the center of the body.

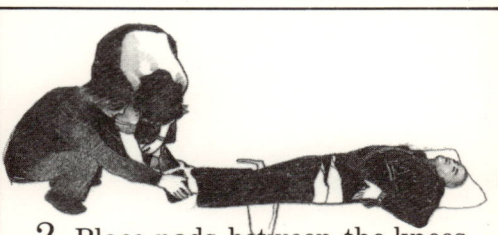

2 Place pads between the knees and ankles and tie the feet with a figure-eight bandage.

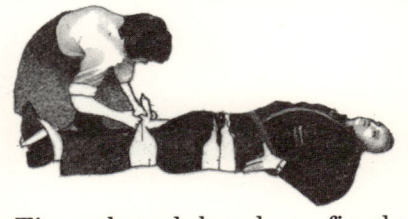

3 Tie a broad bandage firmly round the knees and move the casualty *only on a stretcher*.

Broken Bones/Collarbone

The most common cause of fracture of the collarbone is a fall on the outstretched arm or onto the point of the shoulder. The symptoms are pain and an inability to use the arm on the injured side. You will be able to see, or feel, swelling or the unnatural set of the bones beneath the skin. The casualty will be able to relieve the pain to some extent by inclining the head toward the injured side, so reducing the natural pull of the muscles, and by supporting the weight of the arm.

Action details

1 The casualty should be seated, head inclined and supporting the arm.

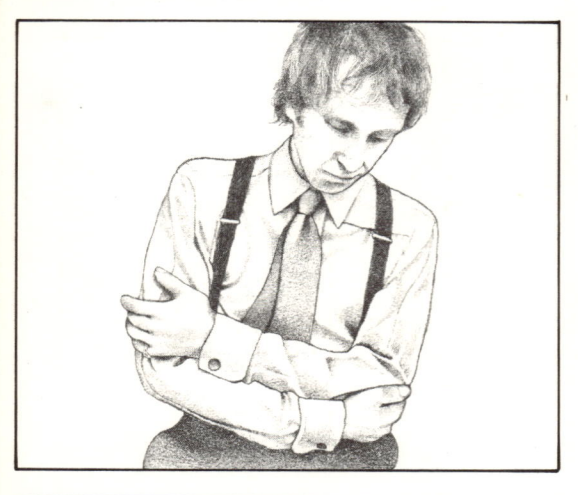

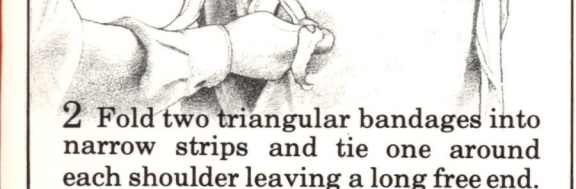

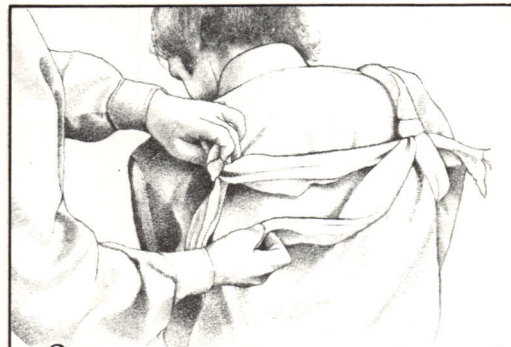

2 Fold two triangular bandages into narrow strips and tie one around each shoulder leaving a long free end.

3 Take each of the long free ends, pass them across the casualty's back and beneath the fixed portions.

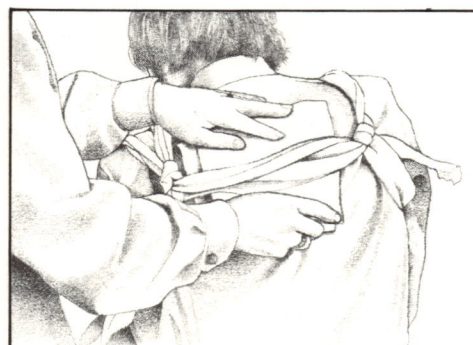

4 Place a soft pad (folded bandage, scarf or sweater) between the shoulder blades and under the bandages.

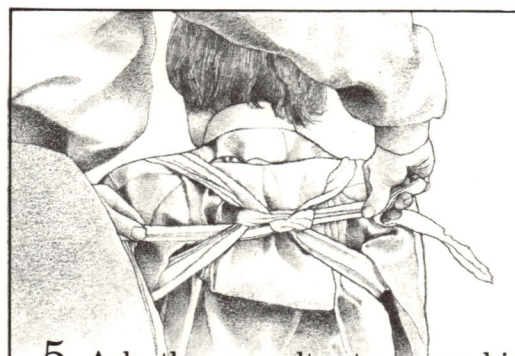

5 Ask the casualty to press his shoulders back, then firmly but steadily draw the bandages tight.

Ribs 80/81

When the casualty's shoulders are braced well back, tie off the long ends of the bandage with a square knot over the pad. Place the arm on the injured side in a sling (**p 73**).

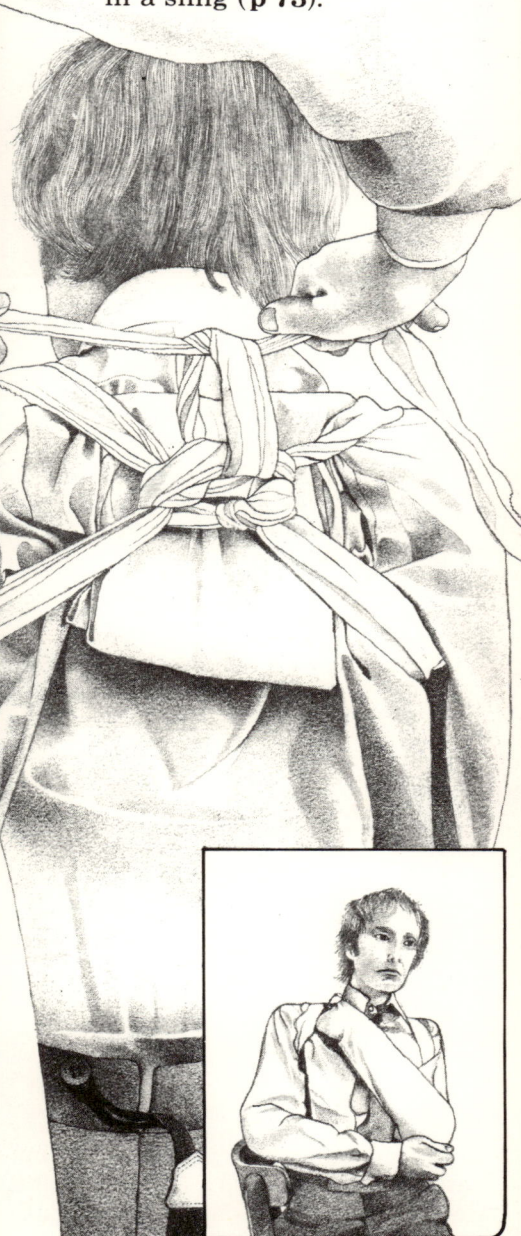

Broken ribs

Symptoms are severe pains in the chest, aggravated by coughing or by the patient taking a deep breath.

If broken ribs are suspected and medical help is not available, support the arm on the injured side in a sling (**see pp 72-3**). The casualty may then be moved into a sitting position or may even be able to walk by himself. However, if the injury is severe the condition may be complicated by the broken ends of bones being forced inward, endangering the internal organs. If there is an open chest wound it should be covered with a large clean dressing; the patient should be placed lying down and turned slightly toward the *injured side* of the body.

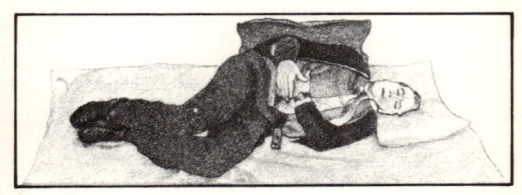

Breastbone

Fracture of the breastbone (sternum) usually results from a crushing force. The condition may be complicated by internal injuries in the chest cavity; the casualty *must* therefore be moved very carefully. Tight clothing should be loosened and the patient made comfortable with head and shoulders supported. Treat for SHOCK (**pp 90-1**).

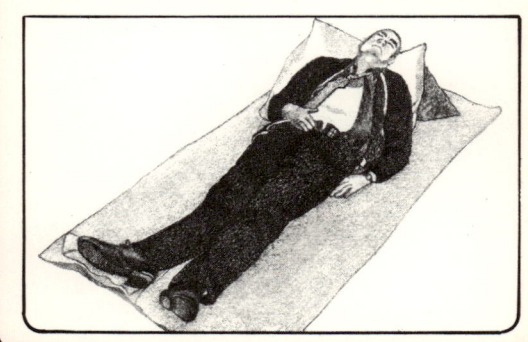

Broken Bones/Jaw

Any injury to the skull or jaw should be treated as potentially serious. Whether caused by striking the head while falling; by a jarring fall onto the feet or base of the spine, or by a direct blow from a falling object, the injury may also cause concussion or even brain damage. In all cases the casualty must be moved only with extreme care, especially if unconscious, and should be taken to a hospital as soon as possible. If the injury is minor, or if there may be a long delay in summoning expert help, take the casualty to a hospital by car. But if the casualty is unconscious...

☎ **Summon an ambulance at once**

Action – fractured jaw

Deal first with the immediate problems of BREATHING STOPPED (ACTION DETAILS **pp 52-7**), BLEEDING (**pp 62-9**) and SHOCK (**pp 90-91**). Loosen all tight clothing and make the casualty as comfortable as possible, either seated or lying down. Remove any broken teeth or dentures and if the casualty is unconscious, ensure that the tongue has not fallen to the back of the throat. Place a soft pad beneath the jaw and bandage as shown. If bandages are not available, improvise. Do not bandage an unconscious or vomiting patient.

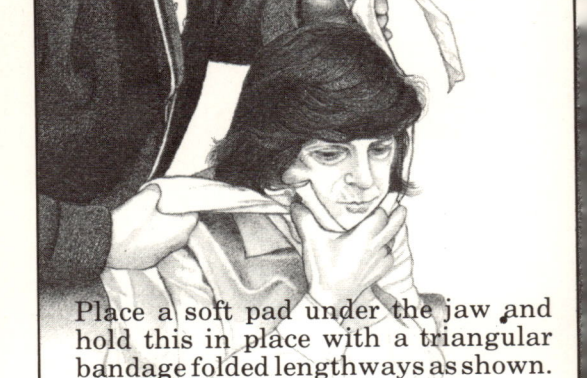

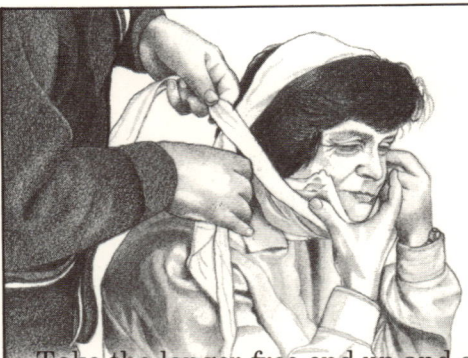

Place a soft pad under the jaw and hold this in place with a triangular bandage folded lengthways as shown.

Take the longer free end up and over the top of the casualty's head to cross the other end above the ear.

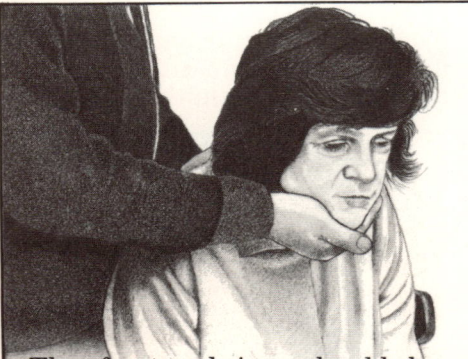

The fractured jaw should be supported by the casualty or a helper to avoid further injury to the mouth.

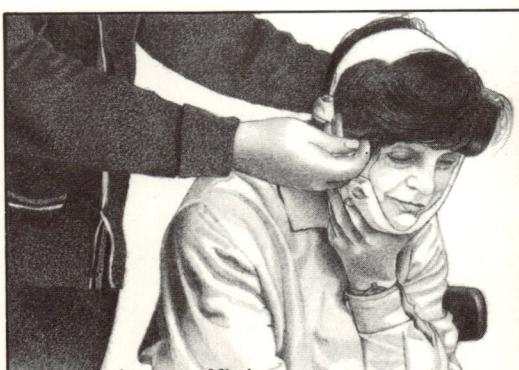

Applying sufficient pressure to support the jaw, take the long end around the head, below the bulge of the skull.

Skull   82/83

Deal first with BREATHING STOPPAGES (**see pp 52-7**) and BLEEDING (**pp 62-9**). Fracture of the skull may be difficult to identify if the scalp is cut or bruised. If in doubt, assume the bone is broken, and handle carefully. In fractures of the side or base of the skull, blood or straw-colored fluid may run from the ear or nose, or into the eye socket.

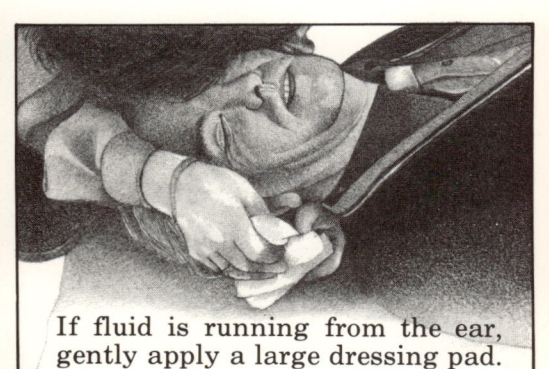

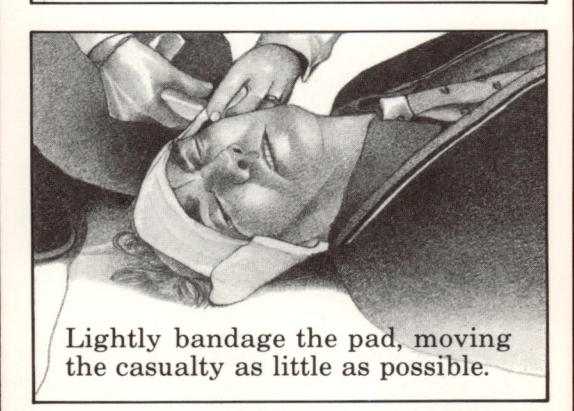

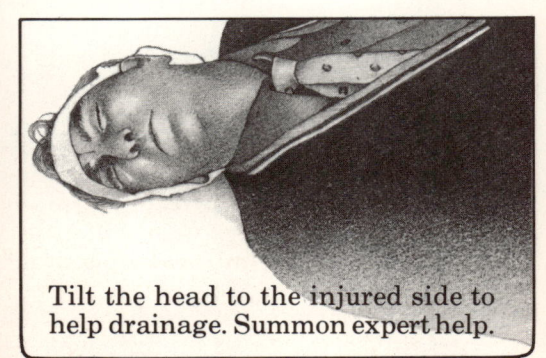

If fluid is running from the ear, gently apply a large dressing pad.

Lightly bandage the pad, moving the casualty as little as possible.

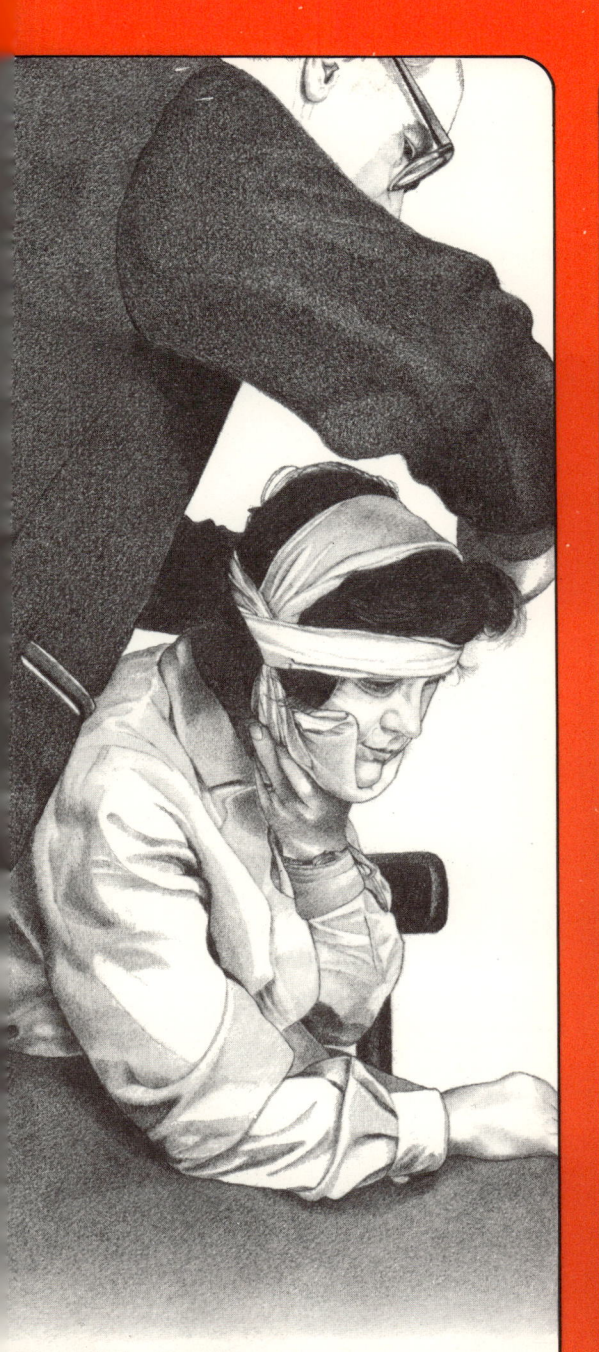

Tilt the head to the injured side to help drainage. Summon expert help.

Tie off the bandage with a square knot above the opposite ear but stay in close attendance and be prepared to remove the bandage if the casualty shows any sign of being sick.

Sprain, Strain and Dislocation

Sprain
A joint is sprained when it is forced beyond its normal range of movement and the ligaments are stretched or torn. The most common site of sprain is the ankle or wrist. *If in doubt, always treat as a fracture.* Similar injury can occur at the knee if the body is violently twisted while the weight is all on one foot. The knee may become locked in the bent position.

Action
KNEE: Support the leg in the most comfortable position and summon an ambulance. If the casualty must be moved, place padding above and below the joint and bandage firmly with an elasticized bandage.
ANKLE: Apply cold compresses to check swelling, pad the joint well and bind firmly with an elasticized bandage figure-eight. If outdoors, *bandage over the boot.*

1 Where possible, elastic bandages should be used to support a sprained knee joint.

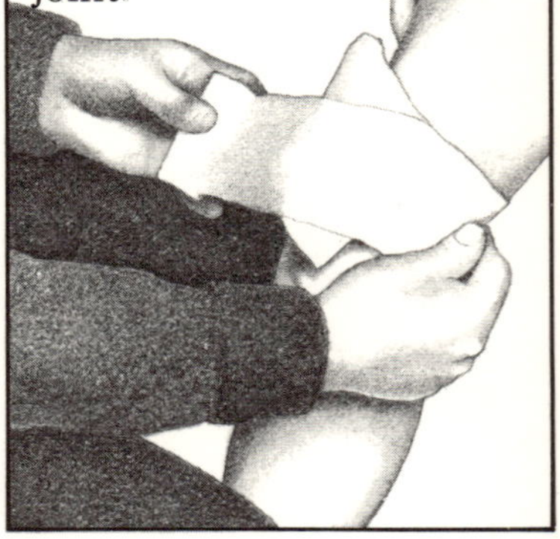

1 Start bandaging with a firm turn round the foot, ensuring that the bandage does not restrict circulation.

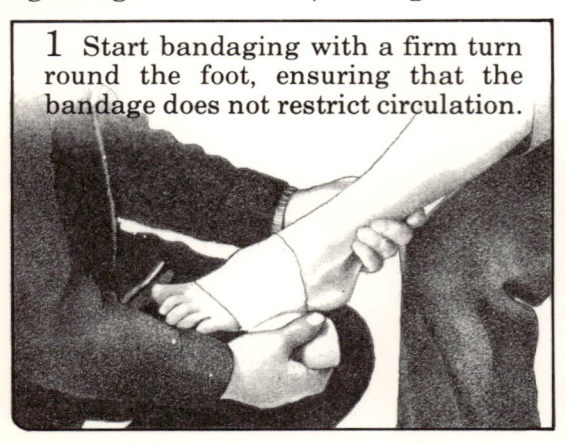

2 Take the bandage obliquely across the top of the foot and round the back of the ankle with firm pressure.

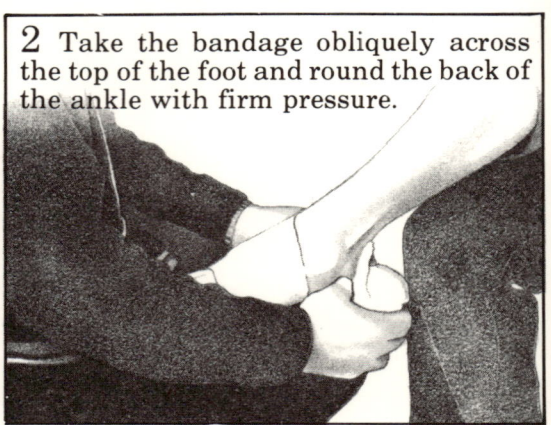

Cramp
This sudden contraction of a muscle or group of muscles can be caused by poor circulation, chilling of the muscles while swimming, or loss of salt or body fluids due to sweating or diarrhea.

Action
The contracted muscle must be stretched, and massaged along its length. If cramp is due to salt deficiency, drink plenty of salted water – using half a teaspoonful of salt to one pint of water.
THIGH: With the casualty seated, support the heel and press down on the knee. 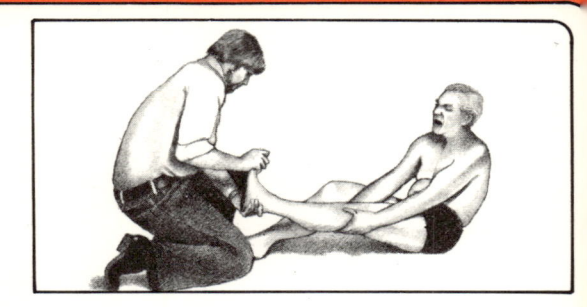
CALF: Straighten the knee and push the toes toward the shin as illustrated.
FOOT: Straighten the toes by pressing upward. Stand on the ball of the foot.
HAND: Uncurl the fingers and massage.

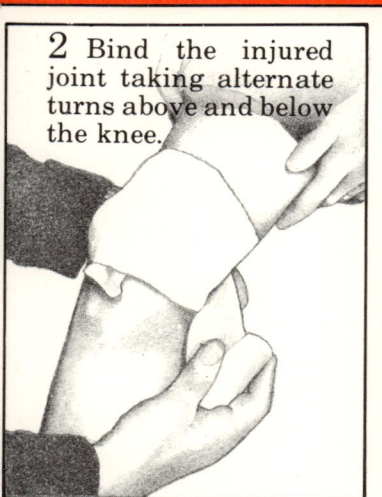

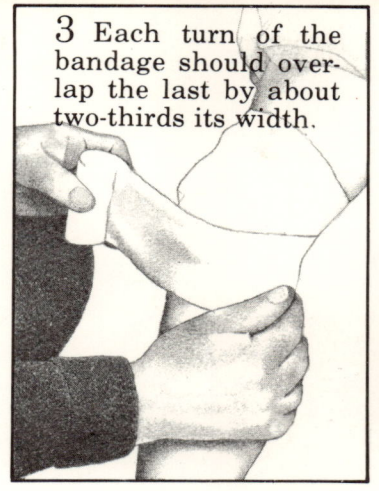

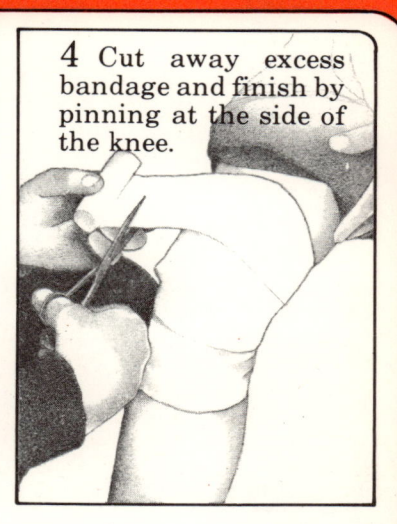

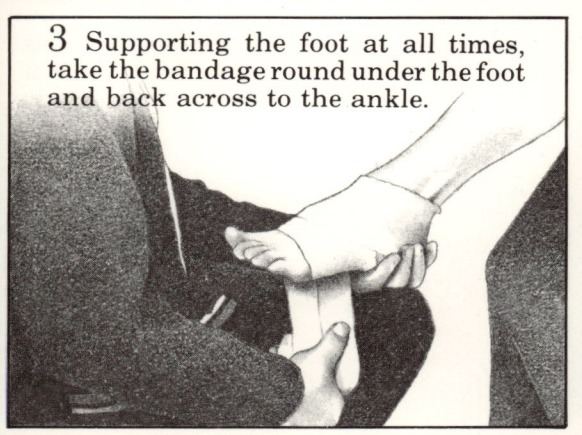

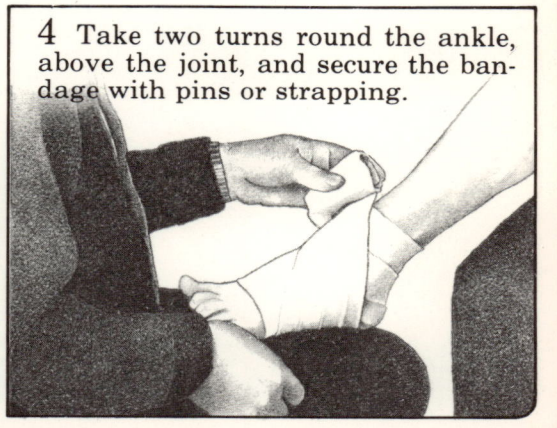

2 Bind the injured joint taking alternate turns above and below the knee.

3 Each turn of the bandage should overlap the last by about two-thirds its width.

4 Cut away excess bandage and finish by pinning at the side of the knee.

3 Supporting the foot at all times, take the bandage round under the foot and back across to the ankle.

4 Take two turns round the ankle, above the joint, and secure the bandage with pins or strapping.

Strain
A strain is the overstretching of a muscle caused by overexertion or by lifting a heavy object. Symptoms are sudden sharp pain at the injury site, followed by swelling and bruising.

Action
The affected muscle must be rested. Support the injured part in the most comfortable position. A cold compress (a cloth soaked and wrung out, renewed as it warms up) will check swelling and bruising. If the pain persists, seek medical attention.

Dislocation
This very painful injury occurs when a twist or severe wrench displaces one or more of the bones at a joint. The usual sites are the shoulder, elbow, fingers and jaw. Dislocation may be complicated by fracture: if in doubt, treat as such. Symptoms are pain, inability to move the injured part, occasionally loss of feeling, and physical deformity.

Action
Use plenty of soft padding around the injured joint and support in the most comfortable position. Seek expert help.

Burns and Scalds

Essential first aid priorities in cases of burning or scalding are: removal of the source of heat; cooling of the skin area affected; action to minimize the effects of shock; and the prevention of infection.

If the victim is a child, or if the burns are deep or extensive...

☎ ***Summon an ambulance immediately***

DO NOT apply cotton, tissues, or anything fluffy to the burned area. Don't apply any ointment, powder, oil, grease, butter or soap – and don't burst any blisters which may form.

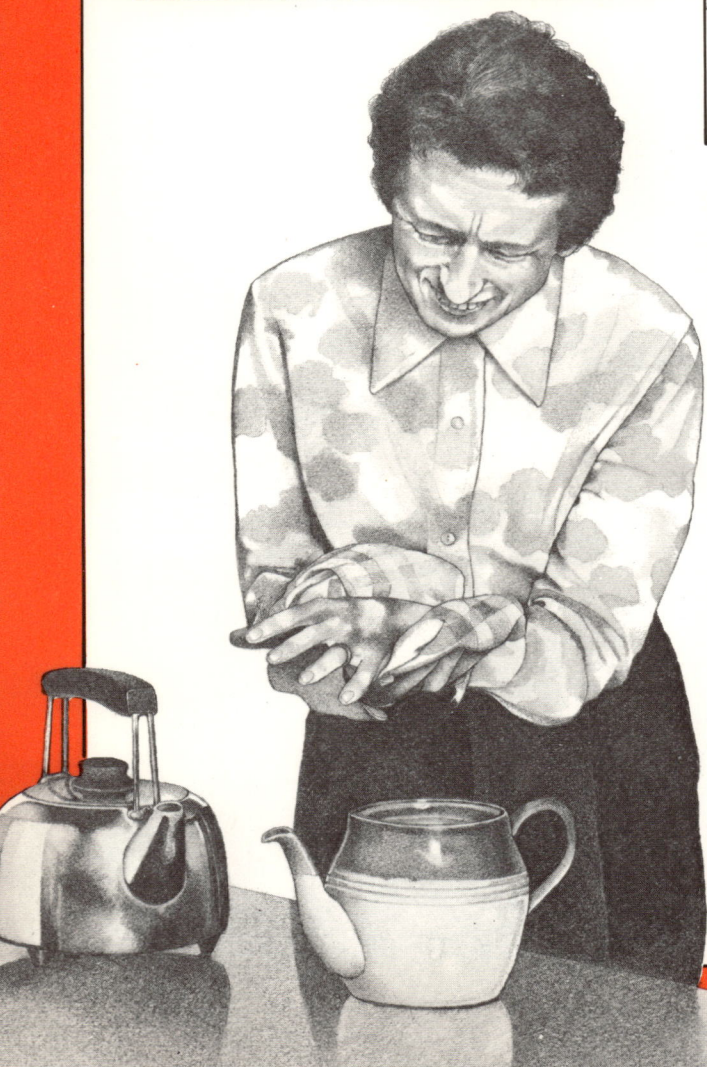

Action details

The burned area should be held under cool, slowly-running water or, if practical, immersed in cool water for about 10 minutes or until the pain subsides. Anything constricting, like rings, bracelets, belts or shoes, should be removed gently before the area begins to swell.

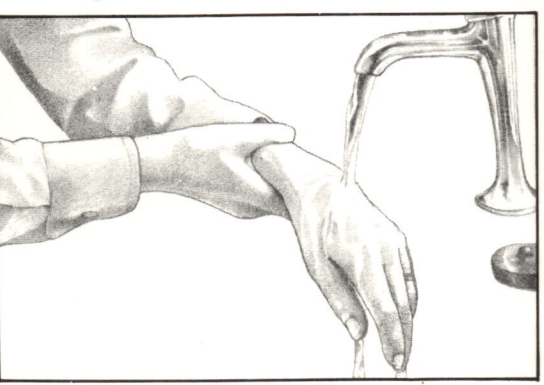

When is help needed?

Small burns, to the hand or fingers for example, can be treated at home but burning fat spilled over several fingers does require medical attention. A common site for a burn is on the gripping surface of the fingers and palm and, while only a small area is involved, expert attention is needed to ensure that no permanent deformity is caused. *In children, and especially babies, even very small burns should receive hospital attention.*

If more than 10 percent of the body is affected (roughly one thigh; lower leg and foot, or head and neck) SHOCK should be expected (ACTION DETAILS **pp 90-91**). The casualty should be taken to a hospital *without delay*. If a car is available, he should be taken straight to a hospital: if he is unconscious, or the burns are extensive, you should call for an ambulance. While waiting for help to arrive, wrap a badly-burned casualty in clean sheets, give small sips of cold water to combat shock, (or moisten the lips with a wet cloth), and keep him calm and reassured.

With a scald, or corrosive chemical burn, the soaked clothing should be removed as quickly as possible – by cutting it away if necessary. Take care not to touch any clothing soaked in a corrosive liquid or you too will receive burns. Cooled dry-burned clothing, however, will have been sterilized by the heat and should be left. Trying to remove it may cause further damage to the skin and will leave the burn more vulnerable to infection.

The aim should be to protect the injury from airborne germs while allowing the evaporation of liquid exuded from the area. Several layers of sterile gauze should be held in place by a bandage or strips of adhesive tape. A clean handkerchief or sheet will serve in an emergency.

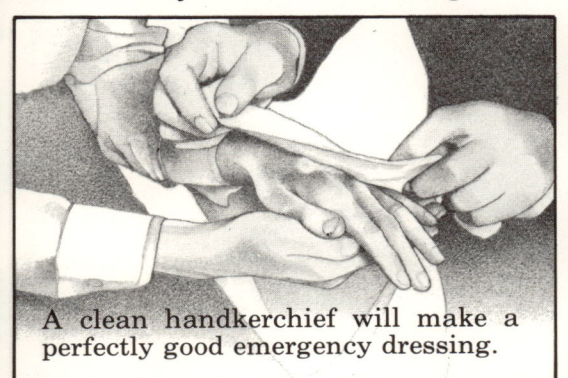

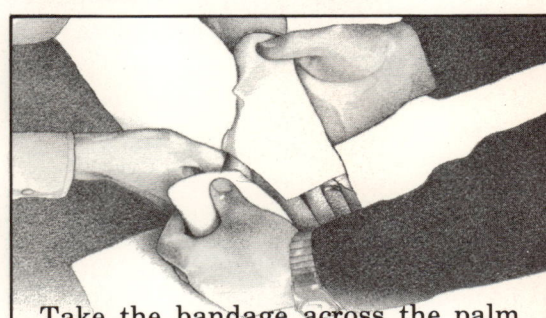

A clean handkerchief will make a perfectly good emergency dressing.

Take the bandage across the palm and between thumb and forefinger.

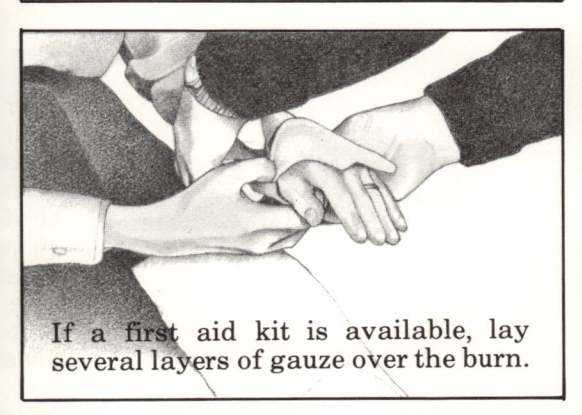

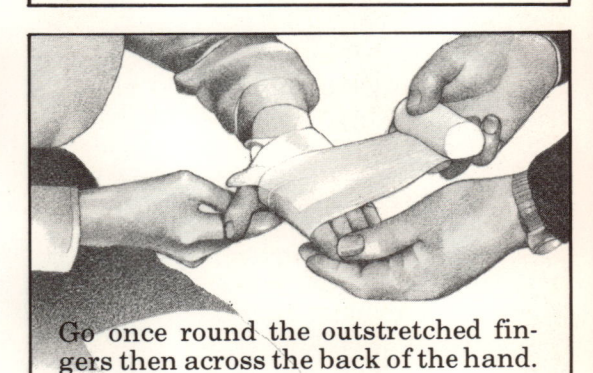

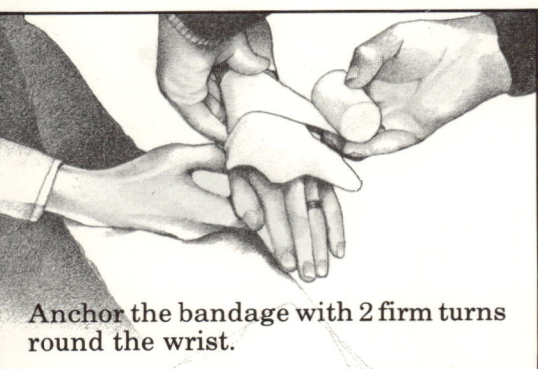

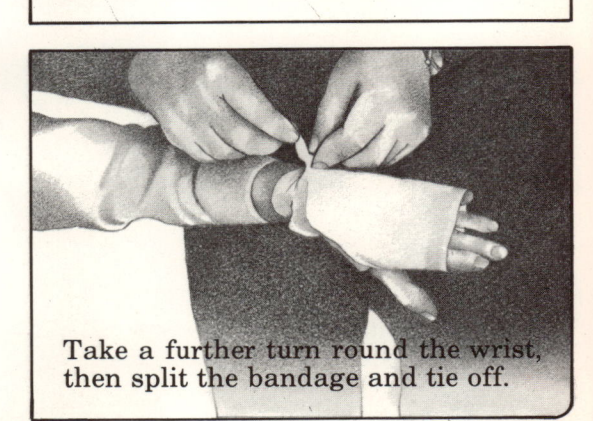

If a first aid kit is available, lay several layers of gauze over the burn.

Go once round the outstretched fingers then across the back of the hand.

Anchor the bandage with 2 firm turns round the wrist.

Take a further turn round the wrist, then split the bandage and tie off.

Poisons and Corrosives

Always keep the telephone number of the State Poison Control Center posted in the medicine chest or near your phone.

☎ *Telephone for an ambulance immediately. If any delay is likely, wrap the casualty up, alert the hospital and drive the casualty there yourself.*

Only when medical assistance is on the way should you attempt any treatment.

Remove any residue of the suspected substance from the mouth – keeping any pills, berries or fluid-soaked swabs. They will greatly assist the doctors in prescribing appropriate treatment. If the victim is conscious, try to find out exactly what has happened – remembering that he may become unconscious at any time.

If the casualty is already unconscious but still breathing, turn him into the RECOVERY POSITION **(see pp 70-71)** so that he cannot suffocate on inhaled vomit. If he is sick, keep the result for hospital analysis, and keep also any bottles or other containers found near the victim.

Many poisons act directly on the breathing mechanism, so be prepared to give ARTIFICIAL RESPIRATION **(see pp 52-7)** and keep going until expert help arrives. The 'kiss of life' is the simplest method but if you think that a powerful poison remains in the mouth, use one of the alternative methods.

If you suspect that the swallowed substance may be corrosive, do not try to clear it from the system. If the casualty is conscious, give drinks of water to dilute the corrosive, but *do not* try to force liquid into the throat of an unconscious person; you will run the risk of choking them.

In any case of suspect poisoning, get the casualty to a hospital as quickly as possible, taking along any container found near the victim, any pills or berries removed from the mouth, or swabs used to clear the mouth.

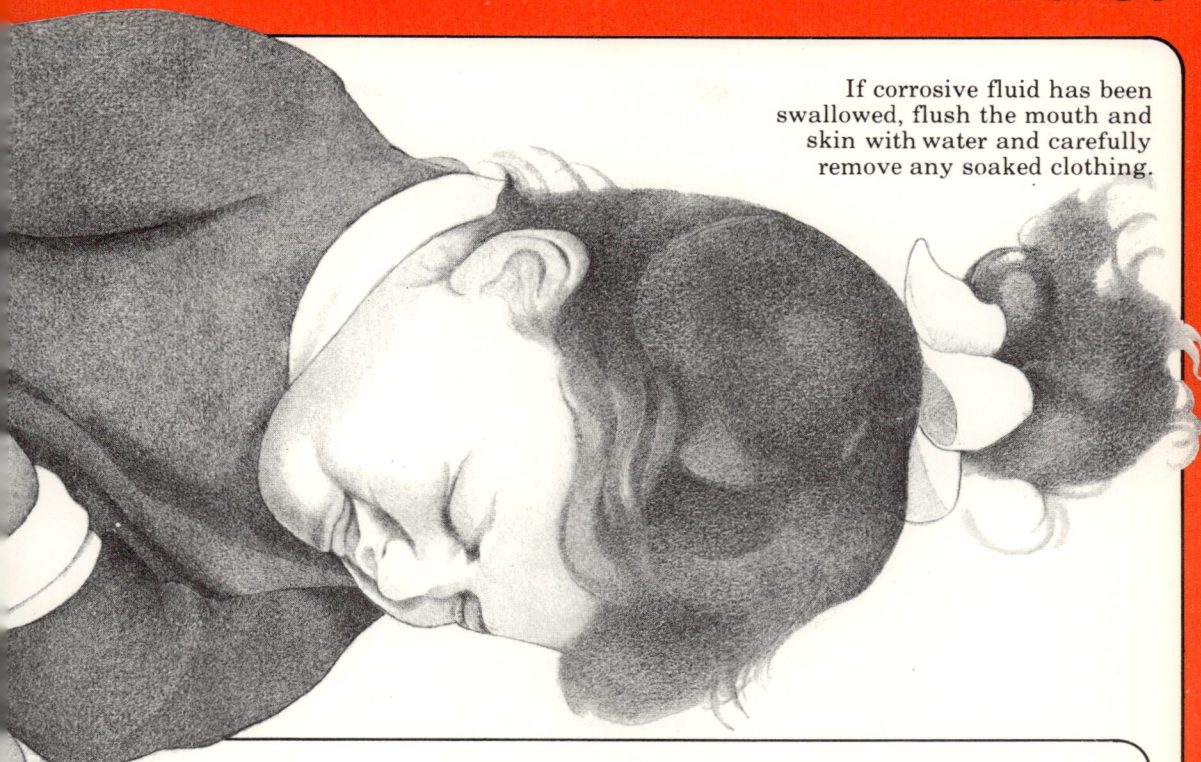

If corrosive fluid has been swallowed, flush the mouth and skin with water and carefully remove any soaked clothing.

The following common household substances have all been responsible for children being rushed to hospitals in urgent need of treatment. All should be kept securely beyond the child's reach.

Adhesives
Alcohol
Aftershave lotion
Air freshener
Ammonia
Antifreeze fluid
Bleach
Brake fluid
Bubble bath
Carpet cleaner
Caustic soda
Cigarettes
Clothing dye
Cosmetics
Detergents
Disinfectants
Dry cleaning fluid
Dry rot preparation
Garden fertilizer
Fire-lighters
Drain cleaners
Furniture polish
Gasoline
Hair dye
Hand cream
Hormone powders
Ink remover
Insecticide
Kerosene
Matches
Medicines
Metal polish
Methanol
Mothballs
Nail polish
Oven cleaner
Paint
Paint stripper
Perfume
Pesticides
Scouring powder
Shampoo
Shoe polish
Silver polish
Suntan lotion
Surgical spirit
Toilet cleaner
Turpentine
Varnish
Washing powder
Washing-up liquid
Weed killer

Any corrosive fluid splashed into the eye must be quickly diluted by flushing the eye with water. Cover the eye with a pad and bandage (**see p 94**) and take the casualty to a hospital without delay.

Shock

Shock is a term used to describe various symptoms that can arise from injury, severe pain or sudden illness. The cause is an inadequate blood supply to the body organs, especially the brain. Shock may be severe enough to be the cause of death so swift emergency action is vitally important, particularly with elderly people.

Signs and symptoms

- pale, clammy skin
- copious sweating
- feeling of giddiness or faintness
- nausea or vomiting
- blurred vision
- clouded consciousness
- anxiety
- thirst
- rapid, shallow breathing
- increased pulse-rate
- weak pulse

Causes

- severe bleeding (internal or external)
- loss of plasma, the liquid part of the blood, likely to occur with burns
- acute heart attack
- abdominal emergencies such as perforation of the stomach or appendix
- Loss of body fluids due to continual vomiting or diarrhea
- reaction in the nervous system due to a sudden emotional disturbance

Action details

The first task is to lay the victim down and deal with the underlying cause: see SEVERE BLEEDING (ACTION DETAILS **pp 62-9**), HEART ATTACK (**pp 60-61**), BROKEN BONES (**pp 72-83**) and BURNS AND SCALDS (**pp 86-7**). Get the casualty to a hospital as quickly as possible: his life may depend on treatment, including blood transfusion.

Moisten the casualty's lips with water if he complains of thirst, *and reassure him*. If unconscious, place him in the RECOVERY POSITION (**See pp 70-1**), otherwise, unless he shows signs of being sick, he should be laid on his back with his head turned to one side and his legs raised. If the chest, stomach or head is injured, the shoulders should be slightly raised.

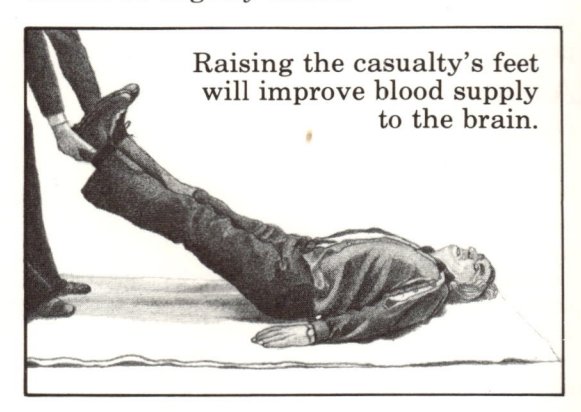

Raising the casualty's feet will improve blood supply to the brain.

While awaiting help, the casualty's feet may be supported on a box.

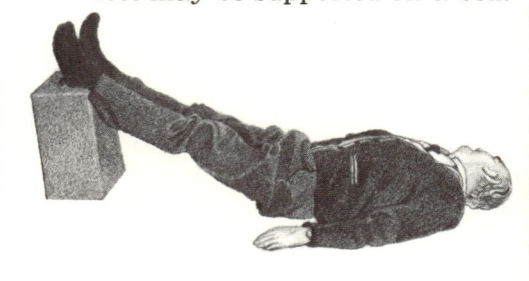

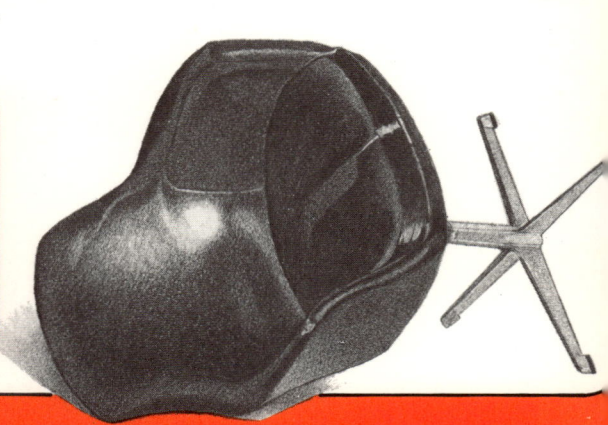

DO NOT

- move the casualty unnecessarily; it often does more harm than good
- overheat him; warming can draw blood away from the vital internal organs
- give him anything to drink; alcohol in particular should be avoided

… fainting

Any of the conditions likely to cause a casualty to suffer from shock may also cause fainting. However, fainting itself may also be a less serious condition and may be caused simply by a sharp, severe pain, by an emotional shock, or by some unpleasant sight such as someone bleeding heavily from a cut.

Often there are early warning signs – swaying, giddiness, pale face or beads of perspiration on the face and neck.

Action details

Urge the sufferer to breathe deeply and to flex the muscles in the legs, thighs and buttocks to help the blood circulate. Loosen any tight clothing and get him to lie down or, if it is easier, to sit down with his head between his knees. Smelling salts are sometimes helpful and small sips of water will help recovery.

If fainting does occur and there is no physical injury, lay the sufferer down in the shade – particularly if the cause is thought to be sunstroke – where there is plenty of fresh air. If he has any difficulty breathing, turn him over into the RECOVERY POSITION (**See pp 70-71**).

As the casualty regains consciousness reassure him and give him small sips of water if requested. If the shock is purely emotional a cup of tea or coffee will be appreciated but on no account should any alcohol be offered. Recovery should be rapid but if not, take the casualty to a hospital without delay.

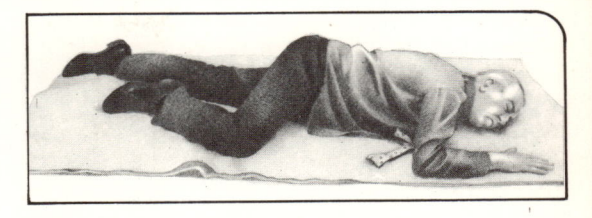

The recovery position (above) should be used if the casualty is unconscious or feels sick; otherwise she should be supported seated with her head down.

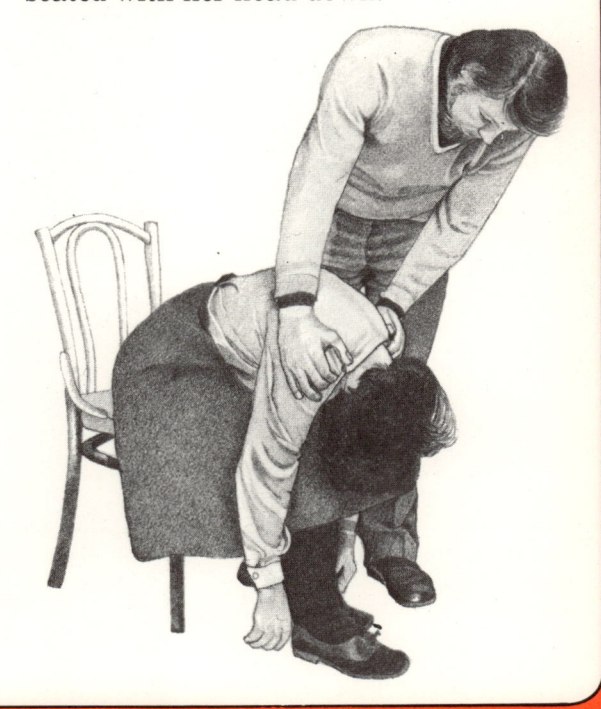

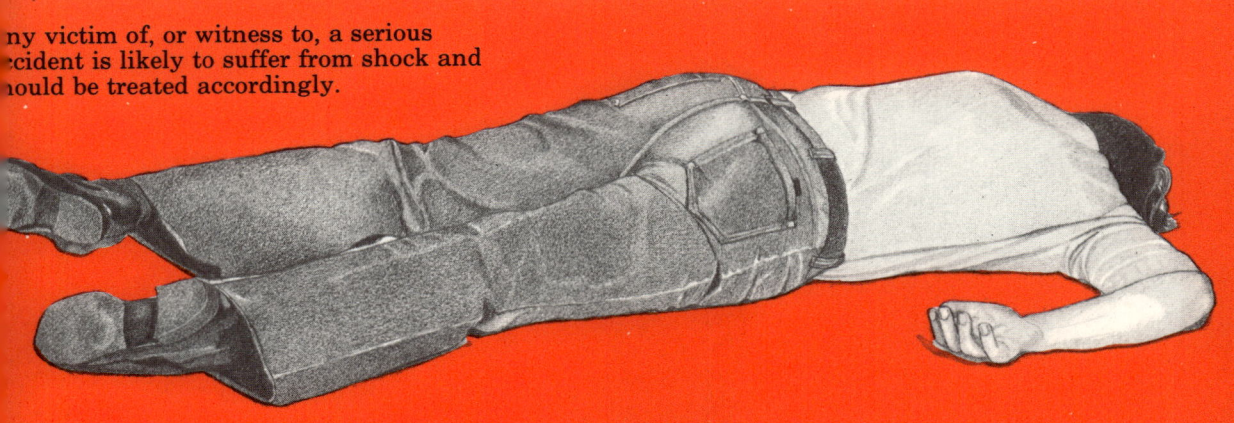

…ny victim of, or witness to, a serious …cident is likely to suffer from shock and …ould be treated accordingly.

Emergency Childbirth

If the process of birth has to be faced without medical attention – don't panic. Remember that it is a natural process.

If you think that the birth process has begun and there is no time to take the mother to a hospital, phone for the midwife or doctor at once. Remain calm, let nature take its course, and don't rush. For the mother it will be an anxious, even frightening time and your own calm will do much to reassure her.

Signs and symptoms of imminent childbirth include low backache, regular contractions in the lower abdomen, a 'show' of bloodstained mucus and sometimes the 'breaking of the waters.'

The mother will want to be away from others, as private as possible. If at home, help her to bed; if in a public place, give her as much privacy as possible. Be firm in sending away curious bystanders.

As soon as you are sure labor has started, begin preparations. If no crib is available, a basket, box or drawer lined with warm blankets and a clean sheet will be quite adequate. Boil a pair of scissors and three nine-inch lengths of string for at least ten minutes to sterilize them.

Scrub your own hands thoroughly, paying attention to the nails, and shake them dry. Boil plenty of water and prepare a surface for the mother to lie on – protecting it with a plastic sheet or with layers of newspaper covered with a clean sheet.

The first stage of labor may last for several hours with contractions becoming stronger, more frequent and more prolonged. During this phase the mother may feel more comfortable and relaxed lying on her side with her legs drawn up slightly. In the second stage, which may last from a few minutes to several hours, the birth is in

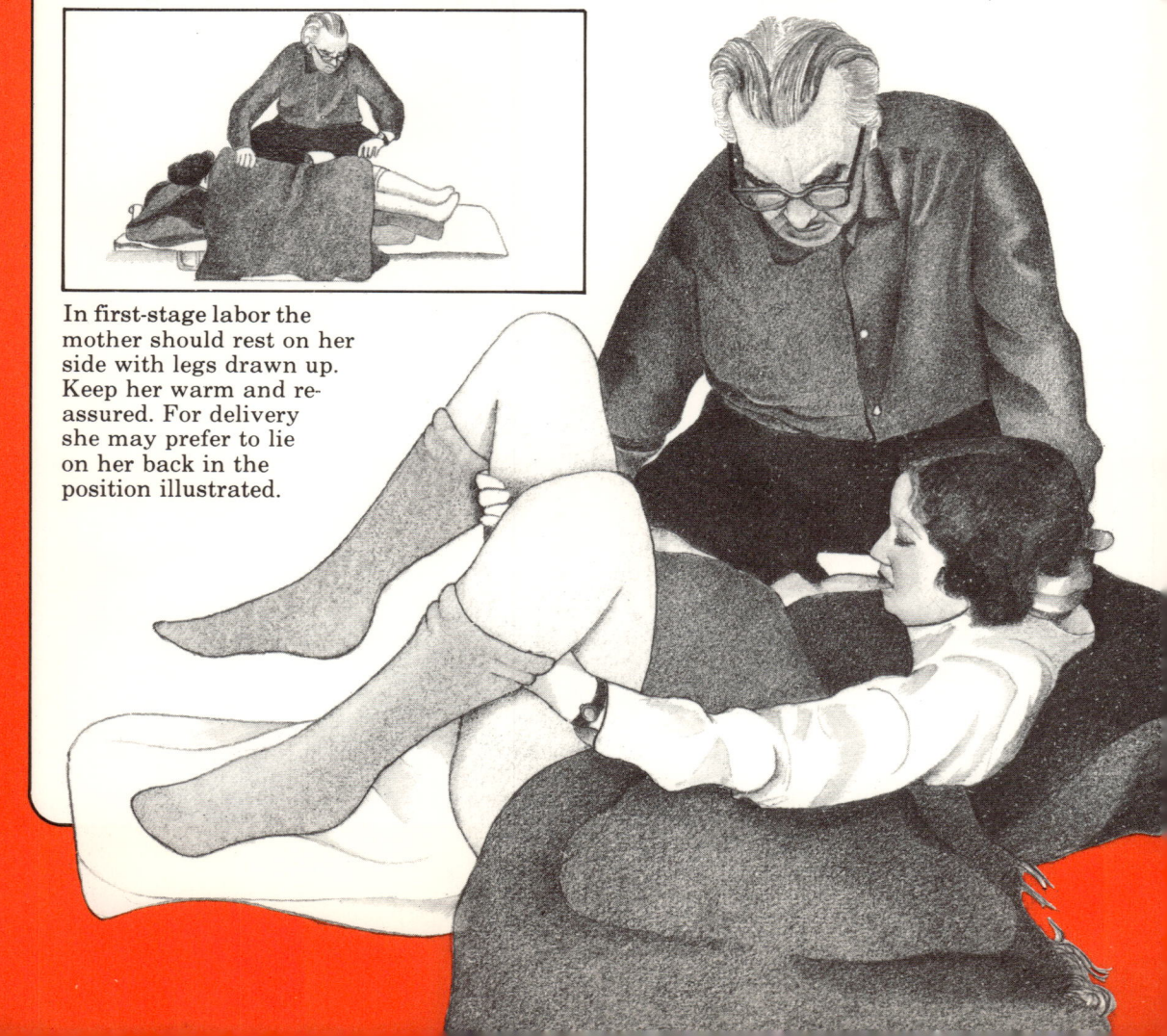

In first-stage labor the mother should rest on her side with legs drawn up. Keep her warm and reassured. For delivery she may prefer to lie on her back in the position illustrated.

progress and will culminate in the baby's arrival. The first sign is the appearance of a bulge between the mother's legs.

Delivery may be carried out with the mother either lying on her back or lying on her left side – whichever she prefers. In either case, ask her to draw up her knees with her heels close to her buttocks.

Ask the mother not to bear down or hold her breath when the contractions come, but to pant rapidly, which helps the baby emerge slowly. On no account pull the baby, cord or afterbirth. Support the baby's head as it emerges but only interfere if the face is covered by a membrane or if the cord is caught round the neck.

When the baby is delivered, wrap a cloth round its slippery ankles and hold it head downward to allow fluid to drain from the nose and mouth. Wipe its face and lay it on its side close to the mother as soon as it has cried and is breathing well. *Do not smack the baby*. If breathing does not start within two minutes, give *very gentle* mouth-to-mouth resuscitation by blowing.

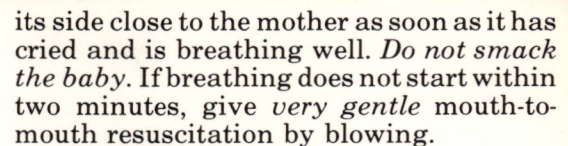

The afterbirth will usually appear spontaneously after ten minutes or more. It should be retained for later examination to determine if it was expelled complete. Only then, and at least ten minutes after the birth, should you cut the cord. First tie the cord very firmly six inches away from the baby's body, and again two inches further away. Cut the cord between the two ties. If the cord is still bleeding after ten minutes, make an additional tie about four inches from the baby's body.

Finally, wash the mother, give her a warm drink and encourage her to sleep. Wrap the baby in a soft towel and place in the improvised crib or next to the mother.

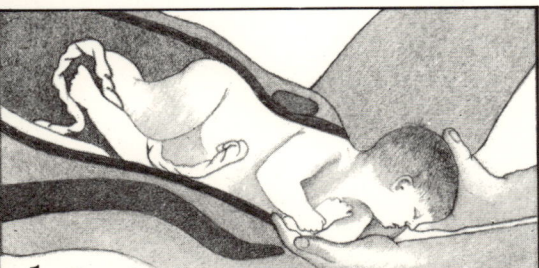

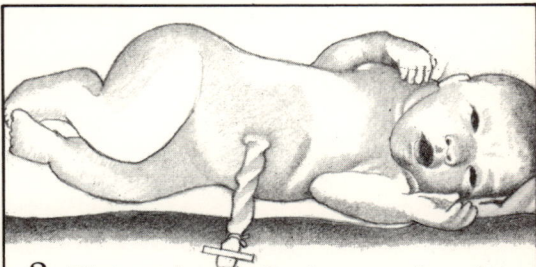

1 Steady the head and shoulders as they slowly emerge but be prepared for the lower body to follow rapidly.

2 Wrap a cloth round the baby's ankles to ensure a safe grip; hold head downward to clear nose and throat.

3 Wait at least 10 minutes after the birth before tying and cutting the cord. If bleeding occurs, see text.

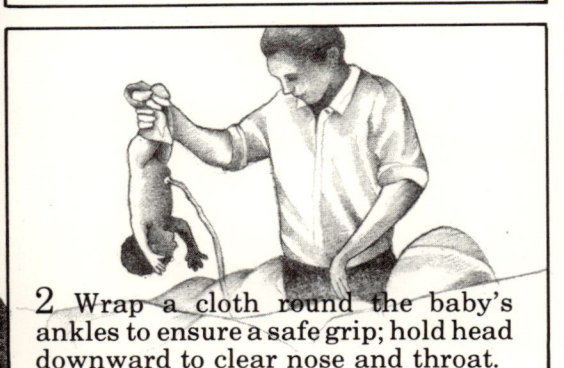

4 Wrap the child in a warm, soft towel and place in the mother's arms. Nothing will help her relax more.

Eye Injuries

If a piece of dirt or dust, an eyelash or a small insect enters the eye, first try to dislodge it by blinking rapidly a few times. Either the movement of the eye-lid or the increased flow from the tear-ducts will usually remove the offending object.

DO NOT attempt to remove any object lying on the front of the eyeball. The transparent part, the cornea, can very easily be damaged by rubbing or scratching.

If the object does not move easily away from the cornea, place a clean pad over the eye, bandage it gently in place, and seek help from a doctor or hospital. If the object lies over the white of the eye you may gently try to remove it using either the moistened corner of a clean handkerchief or a twist of cotton.

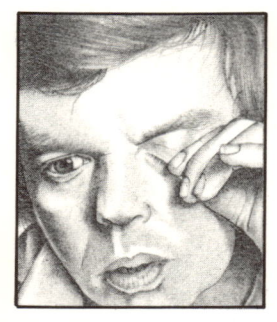

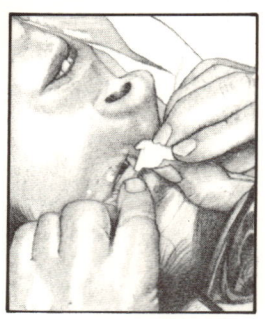

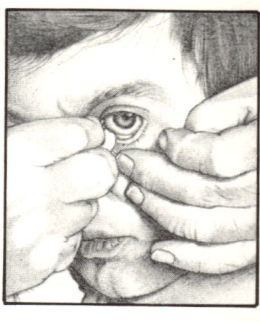

If you cannot see the irritant, gently pull the upper lid over the lower one and let it slide back into place. If this fails, or the object is far beneath the upper or lower lid, ask someone to assist, using a clean swab.

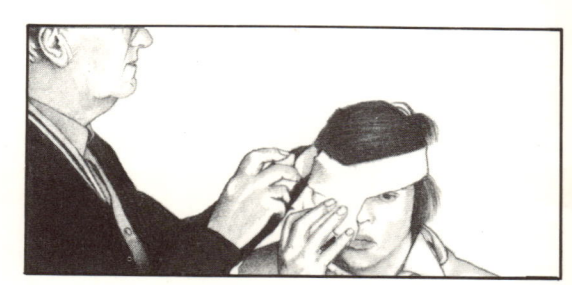

Bandaging the eye

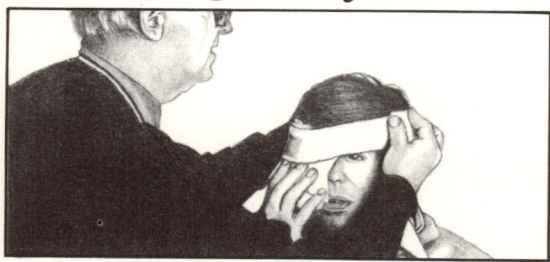

1 If the foreign body cannot be easily removed, place a thick pad of cotton, or a folded handkerchief over the eye.

2 While the casualty holds the pad, take two firm turns round the head to anchor the bandage without pressing on the eye.

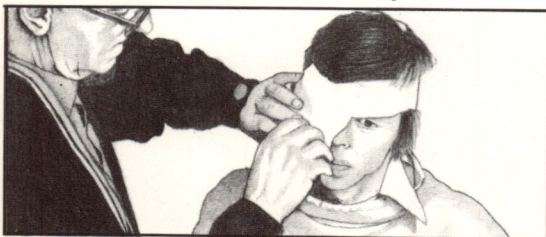

3 On the third turn, take the bandage low round the back of the head, coming up and across the pad but without putting any pressure on the injured eye.

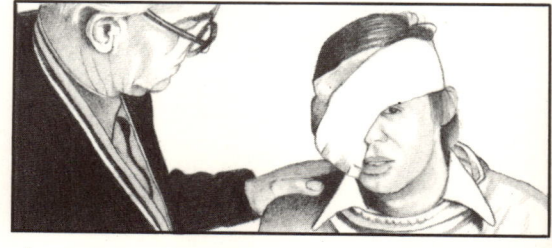

4 Pin the bandage and take the casualty to hospital. *If the particle flew from a saw or sander, seek expert help quickly*; the delicate eyeball may have been penetrated.

Splinters

Splinters are not only painful; if they are not removed quickly, or if the wound is not properly cleaned, they can cause serious infection.

First wash the skin around the splinter with antiseptic, always swabbing away from the injury. If enough of the splinter is projecting from the skin, grasp it with a pair of tweezers and gently pull it out. A smear of antiseptic cream and a small dressing will protect the puncture. If the splinter is deeply embedded, don't 'dig' for it; cleanse the area, apply a clean dressing pad and seek medical help.

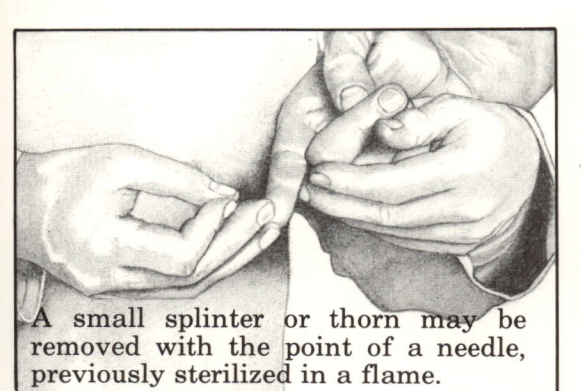

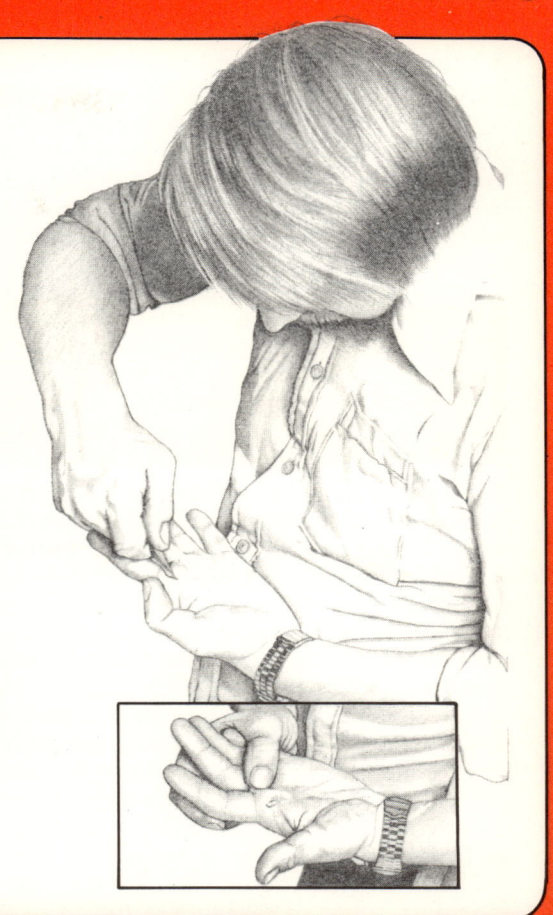

A small splinter or thorn may be removed with the point of a needle, previously sterilized in a flame.

Removing a fish hook

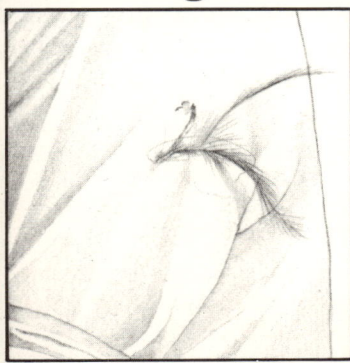

1 If a barbed hook lodges in the arm when casting, do not attempt to pull it out; you will tear the flesh.

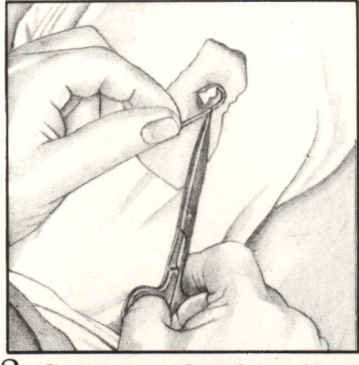

2 Cut away the shirt, line and lure. A small hook may be gently *pushed* through a fold of skin without harm.

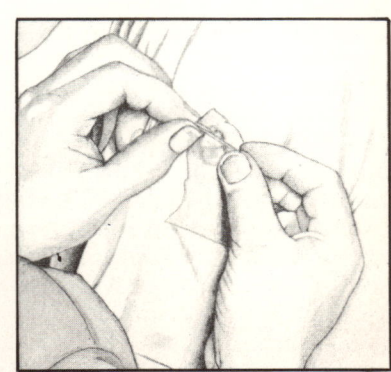

3 A large hook should be pushed through until the barb is clear, then taped to the skin. *Seek expert help.*

Bites and Stings

Although the bites and stings of insects, reptiles, animals and plants can occasionally be serious, their main effect is more often localized pain and inflammation which can easily be relieved. However, if the sufferer shows any signs of undue distress, or experiences difficulty in breathing, this could be due to a severe reaction in the body, in which case treat the victim for SHOCK (ACTION DETAILS **pp 90-91**) and *seek medical attention immediately.*

Insect bites and stings

As the bee's sting is barbed, it is often left behind in the skin and should be carefully removed with tweezers – taking care not to squeeze the poison-sac. Soothing cream, salve, sodium bicarbonate paste or cold compresses will give relief. A wasp sting should be treated with an acid solution such as lemon juice or vinegar. Stings inside the mouth may cause extensive swelling and interfere with breathing. Cold drinks, an ice-cube in the mouth or sodium bicarbonate mouth-washes will give relief but if the casualty is distressed go to a hospital without delay.

There are about 40 known species of scorpion, most of which are found in the USA and Mexico, but only two have fatal stings. Most scorpion stings are little more serious than wasp stings and the initial pain and swelling usually subsides within an hour or two. If it continues, medical attention should be sought.

Insect bites are generally caused by blood-sucking species, notably mosquitoes but also gnats, horseflies, fleas, lice, sandflies and bedbugs. The bites should be bathed with calamine lotion or an antiseptic lotion. Cold compresses or a paste of sodium bicarbonate will also relieve itching. Difficult as it may be, try not to scratch the inflamed area. As with stings, some people may be hypersensitive and medical attention should be given if any strong reaction occurs.

Ticks and leeches are very unpleasant. *Do not* attempt to tear them from the skin;

The bee sting remains in the skin with the poison-sac still attached

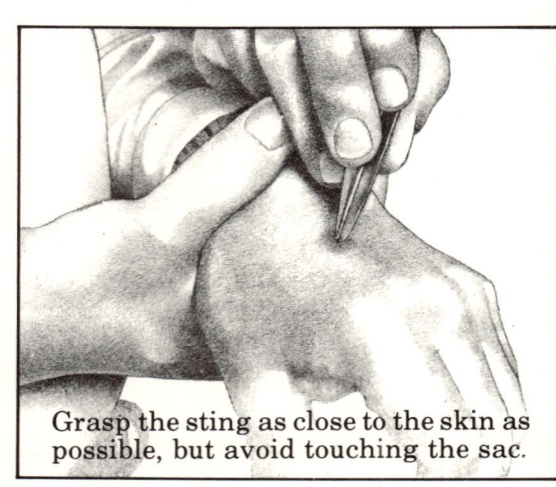

Grasp the sting as close to the skin as possible, but avoid touching the sac.

part of the head may be left in the puncture wound and may cause serious infection.

Applying oil or alcohol, or holding a cigarette near a tick, will cause it to fall off, while salt or a cigarette will have the same effect on a leech. If the wound bleeds profusely, or becomes painfully inflamed, seek medical attention.

Black Widow and Brown House Spider bites are the most common and potentially serious. Tarantulas (in the southwest and Latin America) are more frightening than dangerous. Immobilize the part of the body bitten, keep the victim still and reassured, treat for SHOCK (ACTION DETAILS **pp 90-91**) and seek expert treatment without delay.

Jellyfish stings

A common hazard facing bathers in many parts of the world is that of jellyfish stings which, though usually not very serious, can be painful and spoil the holiday-maker's enjoyment. If jellyfish are present in the water, keep a sharp watch for them and remember that their long tentacles stream out in the current direction: when avoiding a large jellyfish therefore, always remain 'upstream' of the buoyant body-mass. Soothe stings with calamine lotion but if a strong reaction occurs, or if pain and swelling persist, seek expert medical attention (**see also pp 108-109**).

Plant stings

Most plant stings, for example those of the common nettle, are minor irritations which can be relieved by liberal application of calamine lotion, or by rubbing the rash with dock leaves. However, if *any* plant causes a strong reaction, a doctor should be consulted (**see also pp 40-41**).

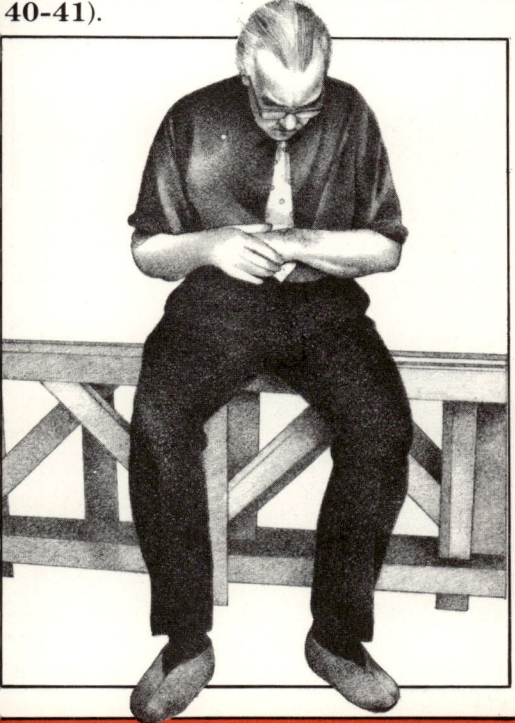

Animal bites

Scratches caused by household pets are not serious but should *always* be carefully disinfected and covered with a dry dressing until fully healed. Deep scratches, and particularly the deep, paired puncture wounds of a dog bite (illustrated below) should, however, invariably be seen by a doctor without delay. Such deep punctures can carry infected saliva far below the skin surface and the doctor may advise anti-tetanus treatment or, in some parts of the world, check for rabies infection.

Snake bites

A snake-bite victim should be calmed and kept quiet to prevent rapid heartbeat and dissemination of the toxin. If the snake *is* poisonous, apply a tourniquet above the wound, make a ⅛ inch 'X' cut over the bite and, *if you have no sores in your mouth*, suck out the venom. Otherwise squeeze it out. Seek help immediately.

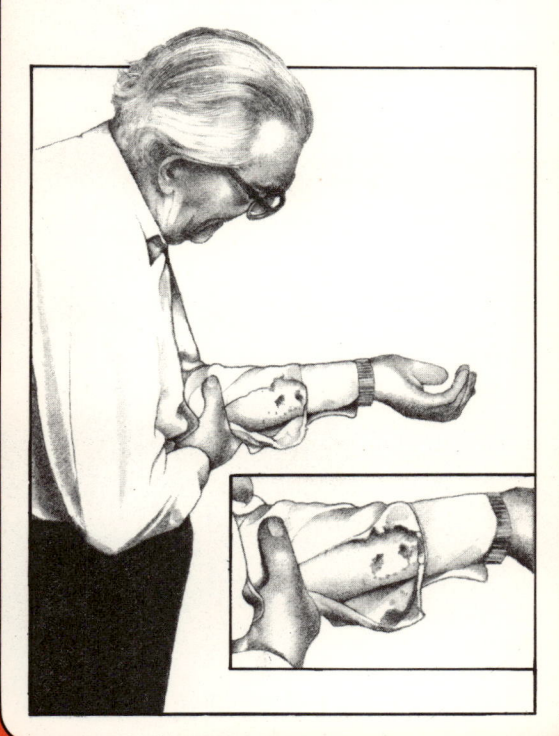

GOING AWAY

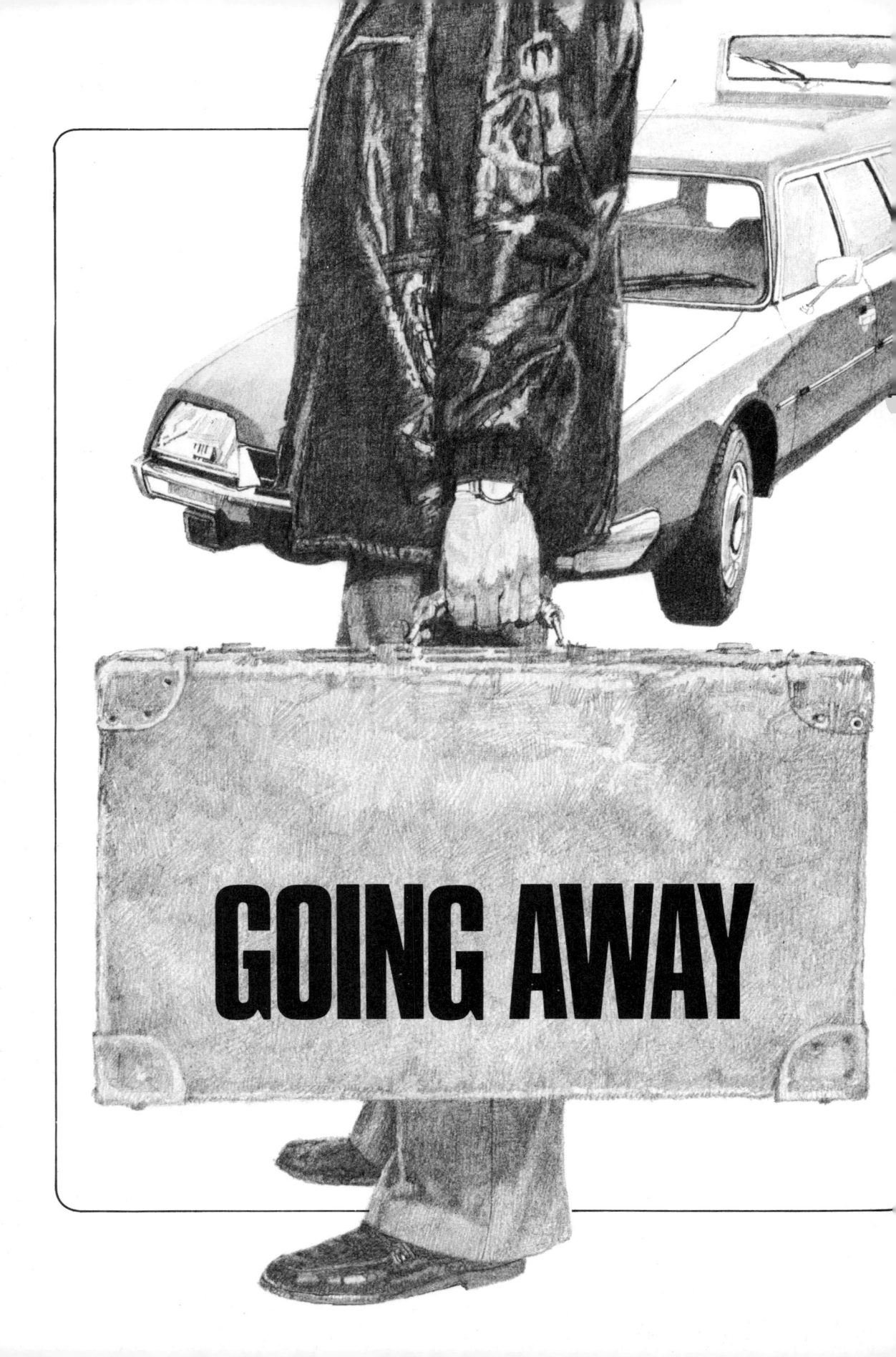

Vacation Preparations

When planning a vacation abroad it is always advisable to take out insurance against illness or accident. Medical care can be very expensive and foreign countries often have very different ways of dealing with illness, both in terms of cost and procedure. Even medical plans may not adequately cover emergencies abroad. Member countries of the European Economic Community have reciprocal arrangements for the treatment and care of their nationals but American travelers in Europe should insure that they have adequate coverage. If medical attention is required, payment will be expected immediately and the tourist in a foreign land, perhaps with no knowledge of the local language and customs, will be in a difficult position without insurance.

The motoring organizations offer a variety of insurance 'packages' covering both medical and accident insurance but if in doubt, an insurance broker or travel agent will be able to give advice.

You should make sure that you are immunized against serious infectious diseases which occur in the countries you intend to visit. Typhoid, tetanus, polio and yellow fever are the most common and some countries insist on immunization against the latter. In some places too you will be advised to take anti-malaria pills. Smallpox vaccination is still required in a number of countries. If it is necessary, be sure to get vaccinated a few days ahead of time to allow yourself time to recover from any possible aftereffects.

Pregnant women, babies and anyone who suffers from eczema should *not* be vaccinated, but seek advice from your doctor or local health officer on all matters of health and foreign travel.

Travellers making long journeys by air, particularly from east to west, may suffer from the effect known as 'jet lag'. Because the usual pattern of sleeping and waking is disturbed, the body's normal daily rhythms of temperature, pulse-rate, excretion and brain activity are also disrupted and it can take several days for the body to adjust to the new cycle. The effects of 'jet lag' can be minimized by getting a good night's sleep before the journey, by drinking plenty of fluid (but ideally avoiding alcoholic drink, which tends to dehydrate the body) and by eating only sparingly during the journey.

Restriction of movement during a long journey, most pronounced in air travel, can cause swelling – particularly of the feet and ankles – so wear light, loose clothing for greater comfort. Include a toilet bag, even a clean shirt, in your cabin baggage; a good wash, and the taste of toothpaste, can do much to relieve the 'stale' feeling at the end of a long flight. It is also advisable to take along some new books or games for young children who quite naturally become very bored if there is little to see or do.

The most common illness abroad is food poisoning caused by eating food contaminated by bacteria. In countries having a hot climate and generally low standards of hygiene, all drinking water must be boiled before use, or sterilized with water purifying tablets. In many areas it is safer and more convenient to drink mineral water instead. Milk too should always be boiled and all fresh fruit should be either peeled or thoroughly washed in purified water. Shellfish is a very common source of food poisoning so take advice from the local residents or others on vacation before being too adventurous. Ask your doctor's advice on a good remedy to take with you for treatment of diarrhea; most attacks are mild and can easily be relieved but, if the complaint persists for several days, or the patient becomes badly dehydrated, seek medical advice promptly.

Automobile Accidents

The tragic toll of death and serious injury on the roads could certainly be reduced by more careful driving, better maintenance of vehicles and the wearing of seat belts: but countless more lives could be saved if only more people knew the correct procedures and priorities to be followed at the scene of a road accident. There is much that can be done within the first few minutes of an accident happening – prompt action that can mean the difference between life and death to an injured person.

It is vital, for instance, to ensure that no more vehicles pile into those already involved. First action should therefore be to warn motorists approaching from both sides. Place warning flares in the road, about 200 yards either side of the scene; enlist helpers to flag down approaching vehicles or park cars with headlights on high beam, hazard lights flashing. At night, the helper should wear light clothing for their own safety – and wave lights or anything light colored and eye-catching.

Quickly survey the scene, noting all relevant details, so that the next car you stop can summon the most effective help.

☎ *He should make for the nearest telephone and call for the police and ambulance services, giving exact location, number of cars involved, estimated number of casualties and severity of injuries, and whether cutting or lifting gear is required.*

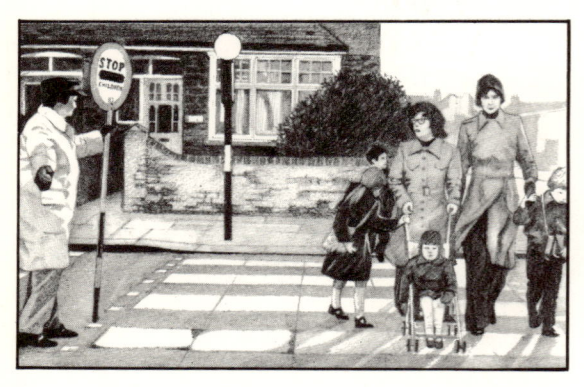

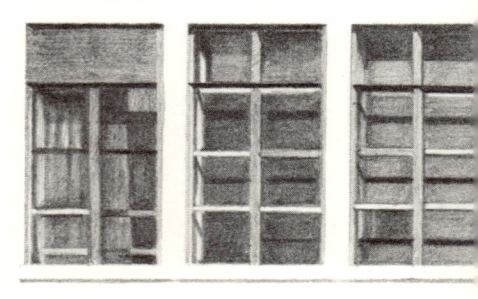

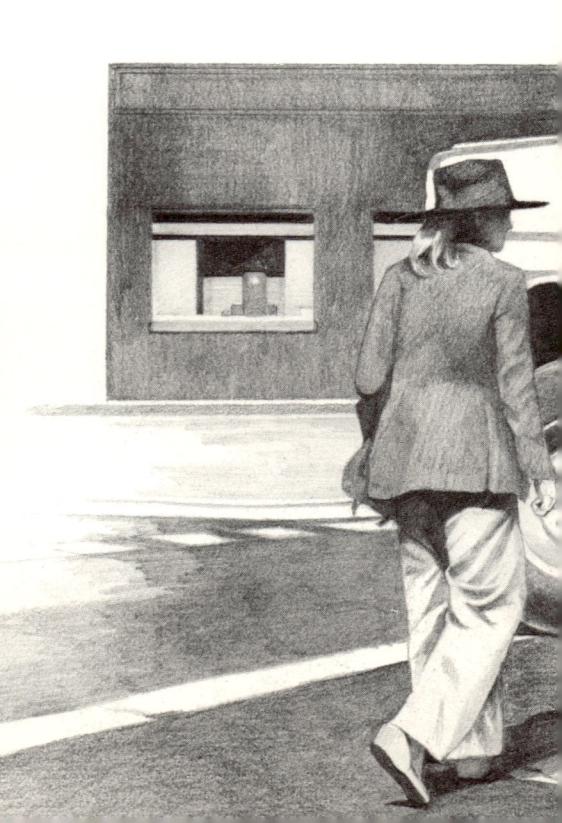

Common sense and constant awareness are the key factors in road safety. Pedestrians – especially children – should always use controlled crossings; all road users must be alert to pedestrians stepping out from behind obstructions, and great care is needed wherever large vehicles are maneuvering.

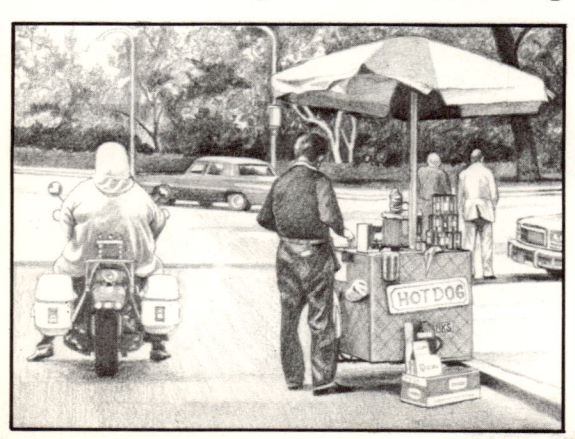

Examine the victims quickly but thoroughly for immediate crises – BREATHING STOPPED (ACTION DETAILS pp 52-7), HEART STOPPED (pp 58-9), BLEEDING (pp 62-9) and then for BROKEN BONES (pp 72-83), BURNS (pp 86-7) and other injuries. *Stay calm, take charge and organize*. Delegate helpers to look after the minor injuries and give reassurance while you, and any other 'informed' helpers, give life-saving first aid to those with more serious injuries. Ask someone to *search* for passengers – particularly children – who may have been thrown clear.

Small fires should be attacked quickly – with extinguishers, coats or by throwing earth on them, but get everyone clear if a fire threatens to engulf a gas tank. To minimize the fire risk, switch off all car engines and lights at the crash, and ensure that nobody tries to light a cigarette.

Do not move a casualty unless he is in danger from fire, or has stopped breathing and you cannot carry out resuscitation where he is. If it *is* necessary to move someone, get help so that all parts of the body can be supported, in case the spine is injured. If a casualty is slumped forward and you suspect his neck may be broken, fold a newspaper into a three-inch band and use as an emergency support collar.

Too many road-crash victims die simply due to obstructed breathing. Check all unconscious casualties immediately, and follow the procedure described on pp 70-71.

While waiting for the emergency services, keep a careful watch on all casualties and be alert to the onset of SHOCK (pp 90-91) which may sometimes be delayed. Question casualties about their injuries; even if a little unreliable due to the effects of pain or shock, the information could be vital, especially if the victim later loses consciousness.

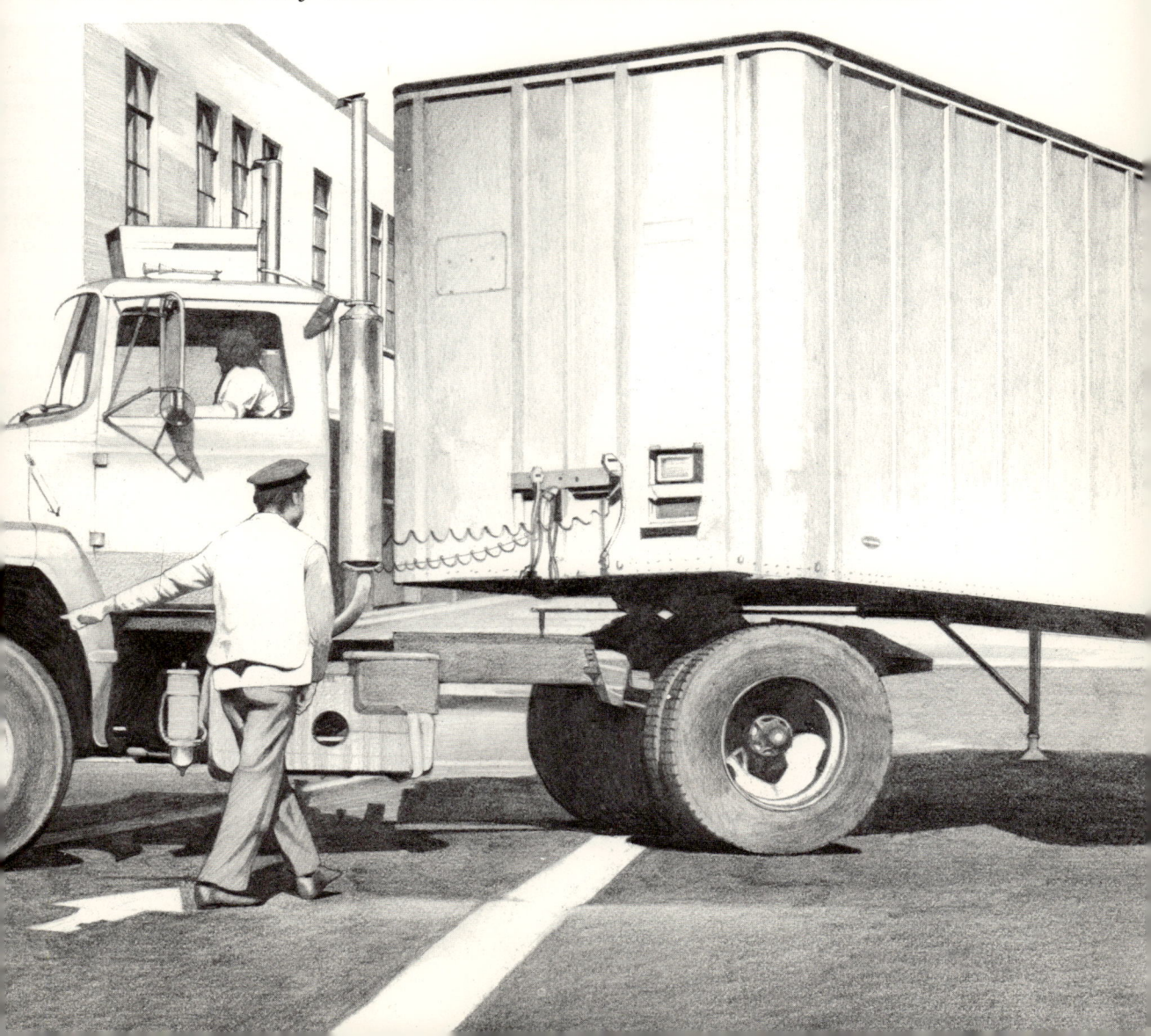

Outdoor Life

Camping is great fun for anyone who likes the freedom of the road, plenty of fresh air and that very special taste of food cooked out in the open. Like many pursuits however, there can be hidden dangers if the simple safety precautions are overlooked.

The biggest danger is from fire. Most tents are highly inflammable because the siliconized waterproofing agent impregnated into the fabric prevents complete fireproofing. There are flame-retardants that can be applied to the inside of the fabric but, obviously, prevention is better than cure. All cooking should be done well away from the sides of the tent and no stove should ever be used inside a small one- or two-man tent.

Gas cooking equipment should be checked regularly to ensure that it is always in good condition. After use, turn off the gas at the cylinder *and* at the burner tap, for in hot weather pressure may build up within the pipe – causing a surge of gas and an unexpected and potentially dangerous spurt of flame when the stove is next lighted.

Pressurized kerosene stoves are popular and economical in use but these too should be handled carefully and well maintained; a faulty jet can lead to erratic burning – a fire risk and a source of dangerous fumes.

Camping sites should always be chosen with care. A site too near the bank of a river or lake, particularly in mountain or hill country, may very quickly become flooded in a heavy rainstorm. Perhaps not dangerous but certainly extremely uncomfortable. Trees provide a pleasant windbreak and a delightful setting, but to camp by a single isolated tree is to increase the risk of lightning strike in stormy weather and also possible damage or injury should dead wood be blown down onto the tent.

Like camping, trailering offers enjoyment, freedom to come and go as you please, and a healthy outdoor life. But again, the major hazard is fire. It is unlikely that a modern trailer would have the stove placed near a curtained window or hanging space but this hazard does occur in many older models.

Another potential danger lies in the synthetic material used in mattresses. If this catches light, even though it burns slowly, copious poisonous fumes are giv[en] off. Cigarettes should never be left burnin[g]

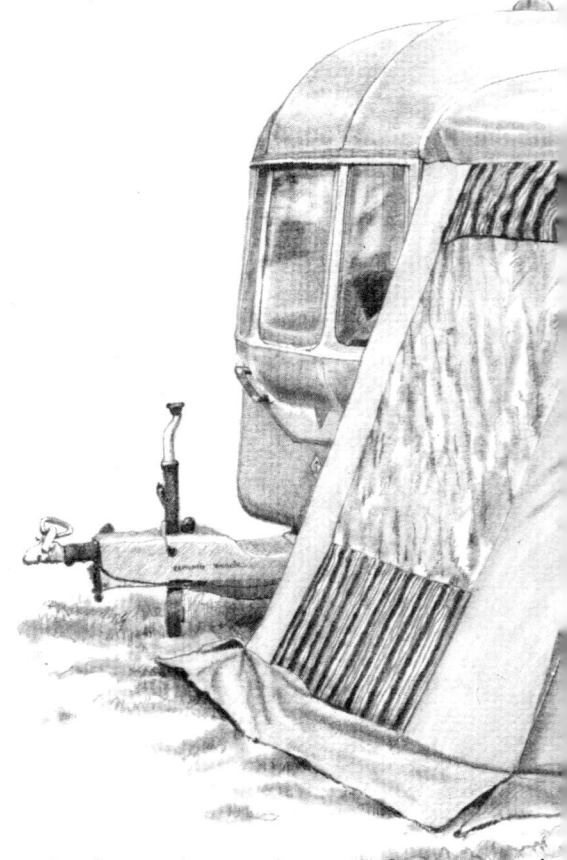

It is advisable not to do any frying insi[de] the trailer but if you do – make sure that t[he] equipment includes an extinguisher of [an] approved design for use both on fats and [in] confined spaces. You will then be able to fa[ce] any potential hazard with confidence. In t[he] event of a fire taking hold, get everyone o[ut] immediately, saving what you can b[ut] taking no risk of being overcome by smoke [or] fumes. Remember that you are likely to [be] some way from a telephone.

Trailer heating should always be by t[he] specially designed convector-type heaters [or] by 'catalytic' heaters which operate on [a] chemical reaction at temperatures no high[er] than 575 degrees Fahrenheit. If in any dou[bt] take expert advice. All gas appliances gi[ve] off carbon dioxide when in use and it [is] therefore essential that the trailer [is] properly ventilated. Again, the mode[rn] vehicle is designed with good ventilation b[ut] many older types are not. Never cover [the] ventilator and do not leave heaters on [all] night unless they are specifically design[ed] for such use and are fitted with fume ven[ts]

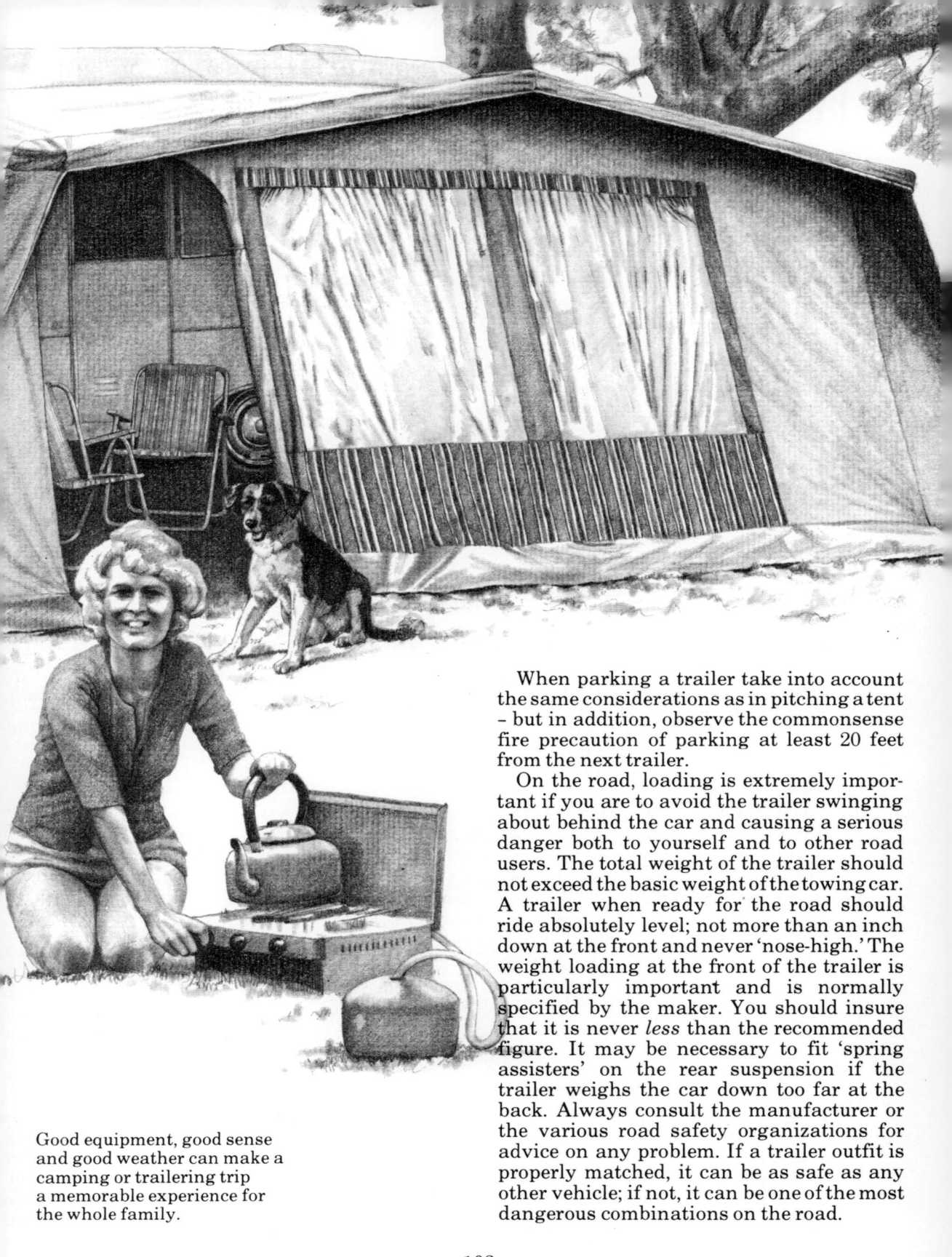

Good equipment, good sense and good sense and good weather can make a camping or trailering trip a memorable experience for the whole family.

When parking a trailer take into account the same considerations as in pitching a tent – but in addition, observe the commonsense fire precaution of parking at least 20 feet from the next trailer.

On the road, loading is extremely important if you are to avoid the trailer swinging about behind the car and causing a serious danger both to yourself and to other road users. The total weight of the trailer should not exceed the basic weight of the towing car. A trailer when ready for the road should ride absolutely level; not more than an inch down at the front and never 'nose-high.' The weight loading at the front of the trailer is particularly important and is normally specified by the maker. You should insure that it is never *less* than the recommended figure. It may be necessary to fit 'spring assisters' on the rear suspension if the trailer weighs the car down too far at the back. Always consult the manufacturer or the various road safety organizations for advice on any problem. If a trailer outfit is properly matched, it can be as safe as any other vehicle; if not, it can be one of the most dangerous combinations on the road.

Hiking and Spelunking

These popular outdoor pursuits can be not only mentally stimulating but also help to promote physical fitness and good health too. But no one should undertake them lightly, for when accidents or emergencies do occur on mountains, on isolated hillsides or in some dark underground cavern, the situation may easily become one of life and death. The secret of enjoyment and safety lies in careful planning and preparation and anyone taking up these activities, particularly climbing and caving, would be best advised to join a recognized club so that he can benefit straight away from the experience of others. Most of the technique of rock climbing, for example, cannot be learned from books; it is best acquired under the watchful eye of an experienced climber.

Plan for safety

There are, however, some general guidelines for safety and survival in the hills. First, always carry a good large-scale map of the area and a compass – and *make sure that you know how to use them properly*. Take along spare warm clothing, particularly gloves, thick socks, woolen hat and spare sweater together with windproof and waterproof outer garments. Take along a whistle, a torch, a small first aid kit and some emergency rations such as chocolate. Let people know *where* you are going and *when* you expect to arrive at your destination. Details should be given to the youth hostel, hotel or guest house, or to the local police station, information center or mountain rescue post. Never go out on mountains or hills alone, unless you are very experienced, and never plan to do too much in a day. Remember that the weather on hills and mountains can change very rapidly, turning what may have been a gentle sun-lit jaunt into a cold, wet nightmare. Take advice: local people are far more likely than you to know when mists are coming.

Safety below ground

The same general 'rules' governing sensible behavior apply also to spelunking, but with a number of additional points. A party should always consist of at least four people, one of them an experienced caver. Every person should carry a cap-lamp and the party should be equipped with emergency lights, food and first aid kit. Never attempt a cave beyond the capability of the least experienced member and remember that the exit from a system takes far more effort, and time, than the entry. Rescue from a cave is often slow, difficult and dangerous.

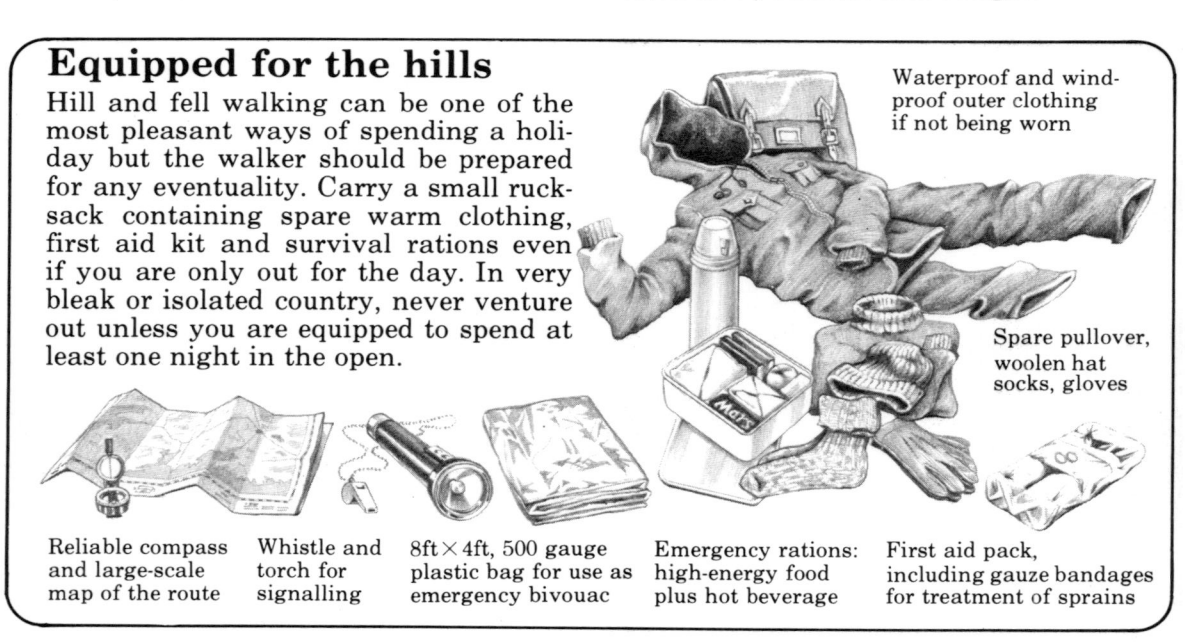

Equipped for the hills

Hill and fell walking can be one of the most pleasant ways of spending a holiday but the walker should be prepared for any eventuality. Carry a small rucksack containing spare warm clothing, first aid kit and survival rations even if you are only out for the day. In very bleak or isolated country, never venture out unless you are equipped to spend at least one night in the open.

Waterproof and windproof outer clothing if not being worn

Spare pullover, woolen hat socks, gloves

Reliable compass and large-scale map of the route

Whistle and torch for signalling

8ft × 4ft, 500 gauge plastic bag for use as emergency bivouac

Emergency rations: high-energy food plus hot beverage

First aid pack, including gauze bandages for treatment of sprains

Wear the correct clothing

Good boots are essential, although they need not be heavy or expensive. They should be broad and have a good heel, to reduce the risks of twisted ankles. The warmth from clothing comes from the insulating layer of air trapped within it. Several layers of light woollen clothing will therefore keep you better protected than a few heavy garments. And to prevent the wet from destroying the insulation, and the wind from whipping away the warmth you need, waterproof and windproof outer garments are essential: a parka is best and, for bad conditions, waterproof overtrousers as well. Also very useful is a large polythene survival bag.

The threat of exposure

The greatest hazard on mountains and hills and in caves is EXPOSURE: cold, wet and windy weather lead, even in the fittest person, to a progressive loss of body heat and deterioration in performance known as HYPOTHERMIA. The warning symptoms are a slowing down of pace or effort, although there are sometimes unexpected bursts of activity. There may be trouble with vision, and stumbling and slurring of speech, together with shivering and tiredness. It is vital to find shelter from the wind for the sufferer and to insulate him against further heat loss until rescue comes. Extra clothing helps and also hot drinks and high energy foods. If the BREATHING STOPS, mouth-to-mouth resuscitation (ACTION DETAILS **pp 52-3**) should be started without delay.

In any accident or illness, give as much first aid as possible and give the International Alpine Distress signal: six blasts on the whistle, or six shouts or torch flashes, repeated at one minute intervals. If help is not immediately available, one – or better still two – of the party should go for help.

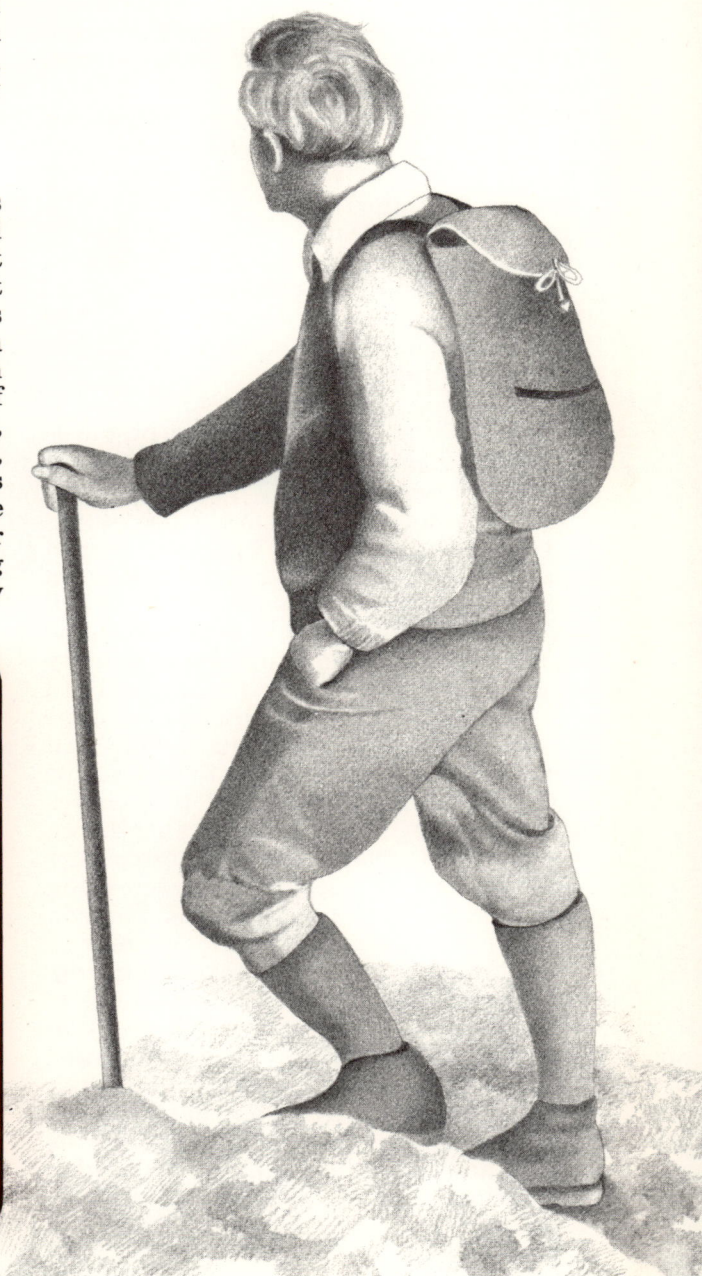

ALWAYS
- ☐ Plan your route in advance
- ☐ Tell someone where you are going and when you will return
- ☐ Carry a map and compass
- ☐ Wear the appropriate clothing
- ☐ Know the emergency procedures

NEVER
- ☐ Go out alone or ill-prepared
- ☐ Ignore local advice
- ☐ Try to do too much in a day
- ☐ Leave an injured companion alone unless it is absolutely necessary. If this *is* so, give him food, protection from exposure, and make sure his location is clearly marked.

Sun and Heat

It takes the body several days to acclimatize to unaccustomed heat, so at the start of a holiday take care not to overexert yourself. Drink plenty of fluids, take extra salt, and do not overindulge in alcoholic drinks. Not taking these simple precautions can result in HEAT EXHAUSTION, the symptoms of which are lethargy, giddiness, headaches and nausea. If this does happen, the patient should rest in a cool room and be given plenty of fluids and extra salt (**see also** under CRAMP, ACTION DETAILS p 84).

Severe or prolonged exposure to heat can result in HEATSTROKE. Symptoms are rapid pulse, hot dry skin, raised temperature and vomiting. Cool the patient by fanning or by spraying with cool water. Once the temperature begins to return to normal, the treatment is the same as for heat exhaustion. Medical attention is advisable in either case – and imperative if, in an extreme case, the patient goes into a coma.

SUNSTROKE is the direct result of overexposure to intense sunlight and produces symptoms similar to those of heat exhaustion or heatstroke.

Mere tanning of the skin is a healthy sign – it is the development of dark pigment deep in the skin which acts as a natural protection against the sun's rays. However, when exposure to strong sunlight is overdone, the result can be painful burning. It is all too easy to underestimate the strength of the sun until it is too late. In a Mediterranean-type climate, never sunbathe for more than half an hour on the first day; less if you are fair-skinned. In the tropics, just 15 minutes should be the maximum. On succeeding days, it should be safe to double the exposure time but take care, use a good sunscreening cream and avoid the midday sun. You *can* buy various vitamin-A and calcium carbonate tablets designed to prevent burning, but there is still some medical debate as to just how effective they are. Calamine lotion is a useful soothing agent if you do get burned and it is far cheaper than many of the after-sun lotions marketed. If severe burning does occur, seek medical attention as quickly as possible and *do not burst any blisters* which may form: you will expose the burn to infection and slow down healing.

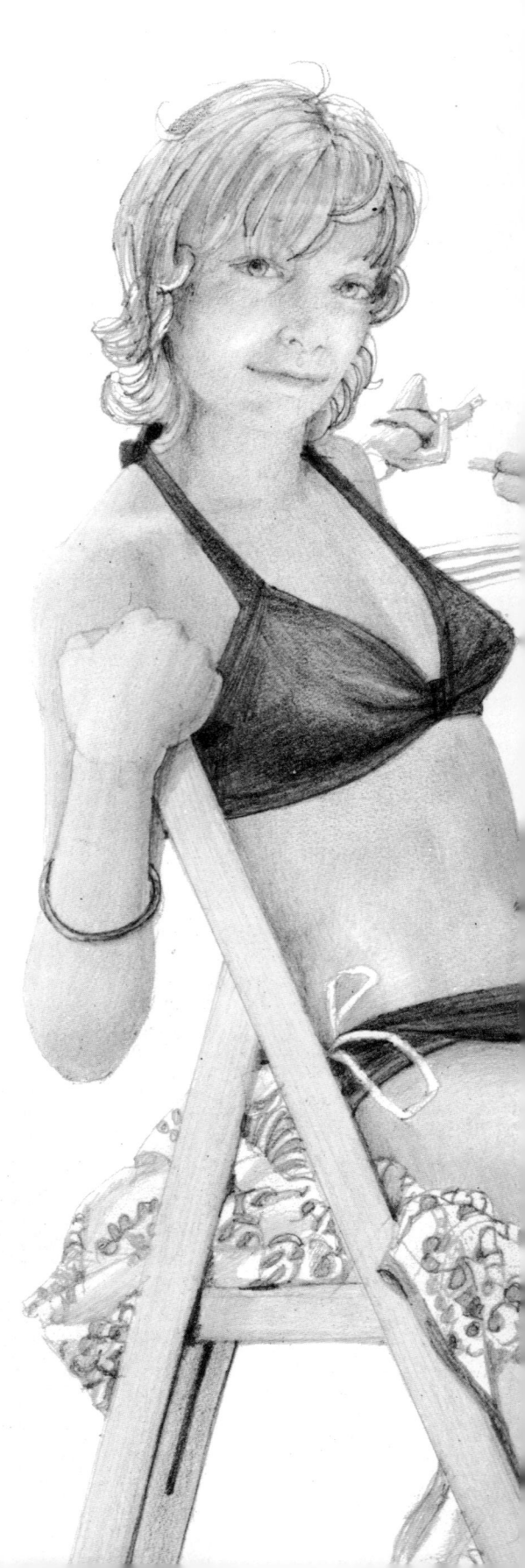

The unsuspected hazard

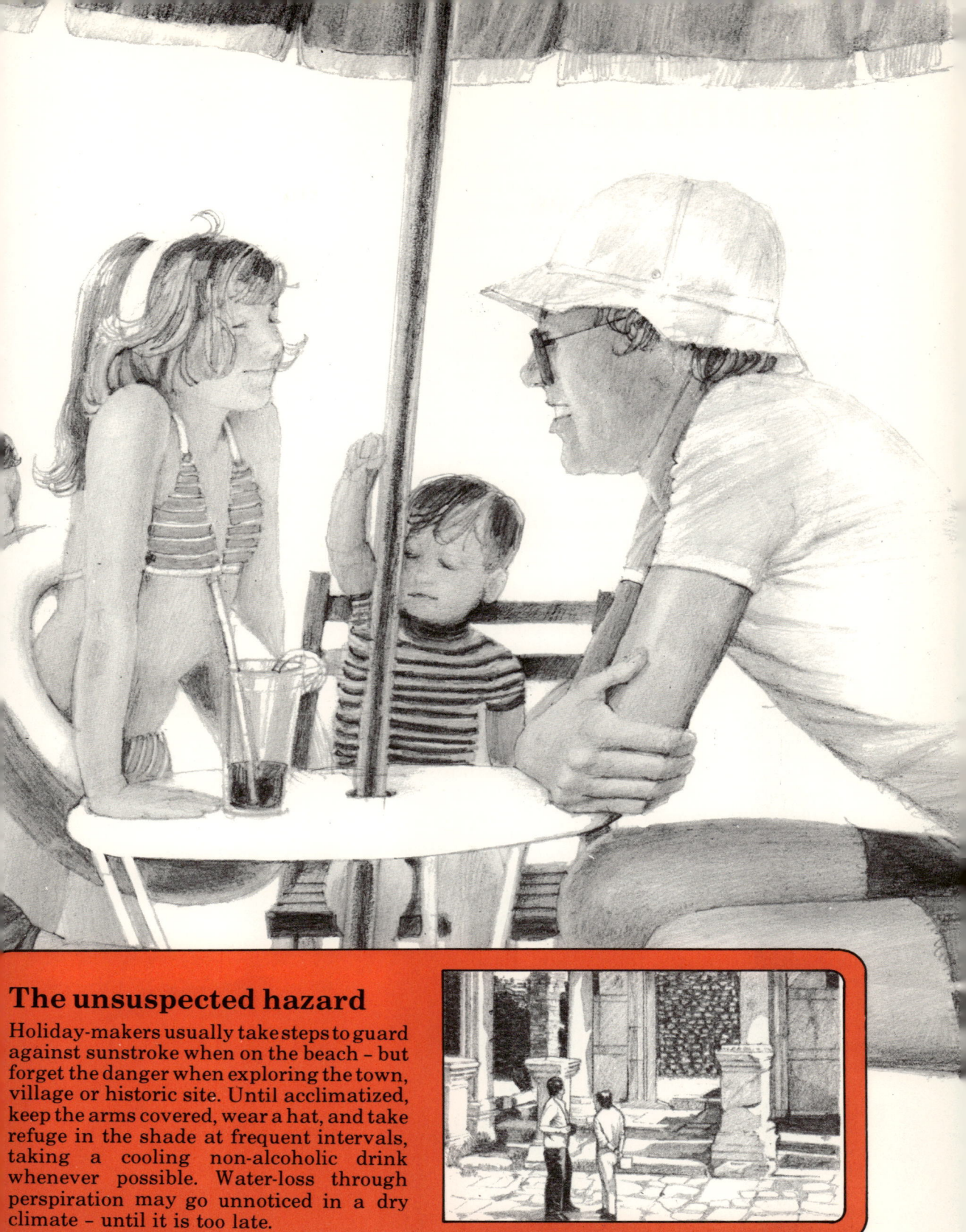

Holiday-makers usually take steps to guard against sunstroke when on the beach – but forget the danger when exploring the town, village or historic site. Until acclimatized, keep the arms covered, wear a hat, and take refuge in the shade at frequent intervals, taking a cooling non-alcoholic drink whenever possible. Water-loss through perspiration may go unnoticed in a dry climate – until it is too late.

Water Sports

The sea does not tolerate fools – and while swimming, surfing, water-skiing and messing about in boats are invigorating and enjoyable holiday activities, all require care if tragic accidents are to be avoided.

Precautions while bathing rely mainly on common sense, but even so, many children and adults die every year by drowning. There is at present no international, unified method of marking unsafe beaches but where warning notices or red flags are displayed, they should be strictly observed. If no such signs are evident, take local advice before taking the plunge; an apparently safe beach may be subject to dangerous currents at some states of the tide.

Chilling of the muscles while swimming can cause cramp. If this happens, stay calm. Try and attract help but continue to use the unaffected limbs to make for shore. Treatment for cramp is described on p 84.

Around European shores, most jellyfish are fairly harmless but if you are stung it is advisable to seek medical attention. First remove any parts of the animal sticking to the skin, making sure that your fingers are well covered with wet sand. Then bathe the affected area with methanol, calamine lotion or soothing cream. The one dangerous species found in European waters is the 'Portuguese Man-of-War,' recognizable by its pale blue buoyant body-mass. The stinging tentacles stick to the skin and cannot be brushed off so the poison capsules should be scraped off the surface using wet sand, after which medical attention should be sought as quickly as possible.

Many more dangerous species are found in northern Australian, Indian and Pacific waters. Some of these have potentially fatal stings and urgent medical attention should always be sought. Also around these shores are found a number of poisonous fish. Some bite and some sting, but in most the venom has a depressant effect on the heart and immediate medical attention is required.

Weaver fish and sea urchins, found around Atlantic and Mediterranean shores, have poisonous spines which can cause painful injuries – usually to the feet. If they are present locally, protective footwear should be worn on the beach *and* in the water.

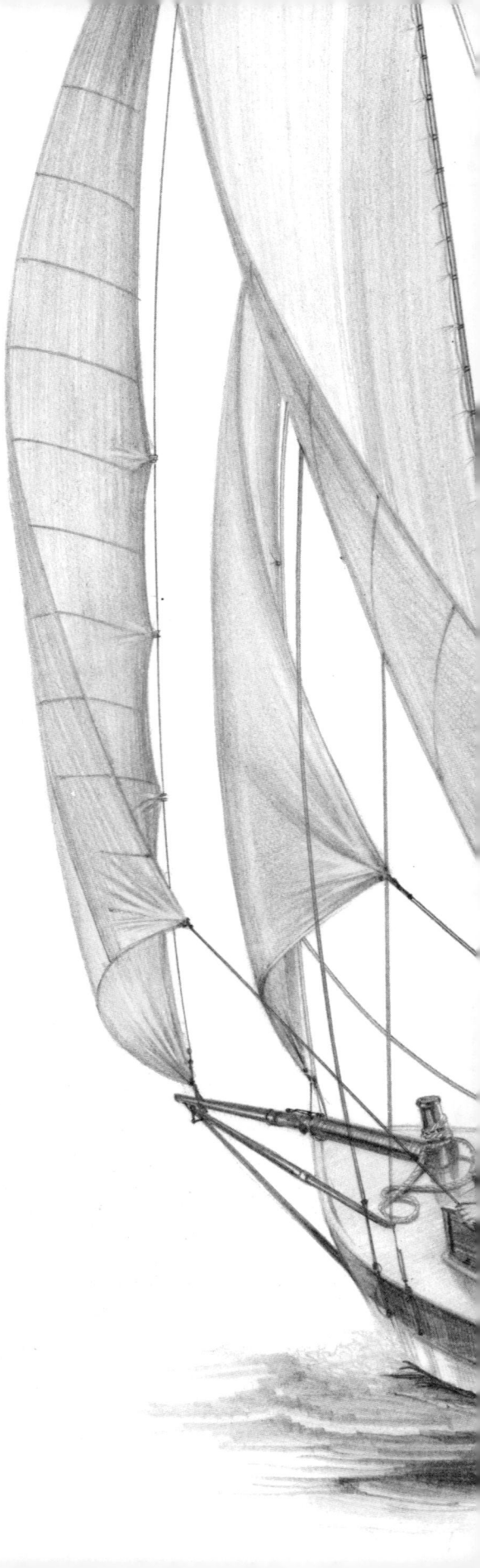

Water-skiing is fast and exhilarating but great care must be taken to avoid injury to bathers.

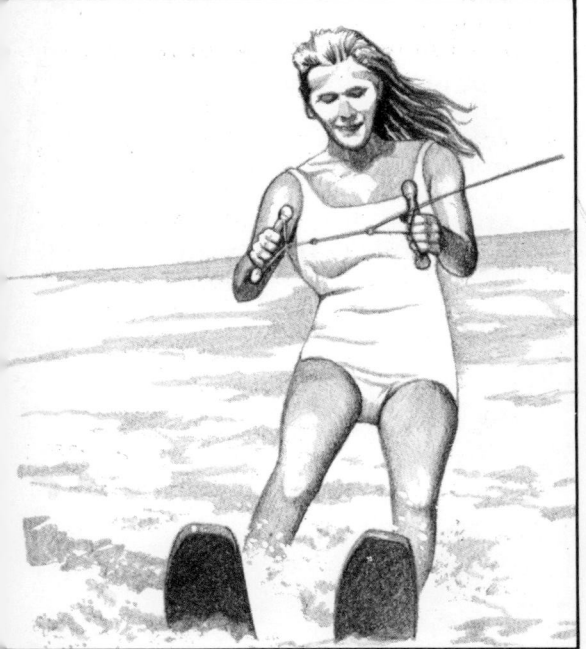

Children *must* be supervised. When playing with floats they can drift, or be blown, out to sea.

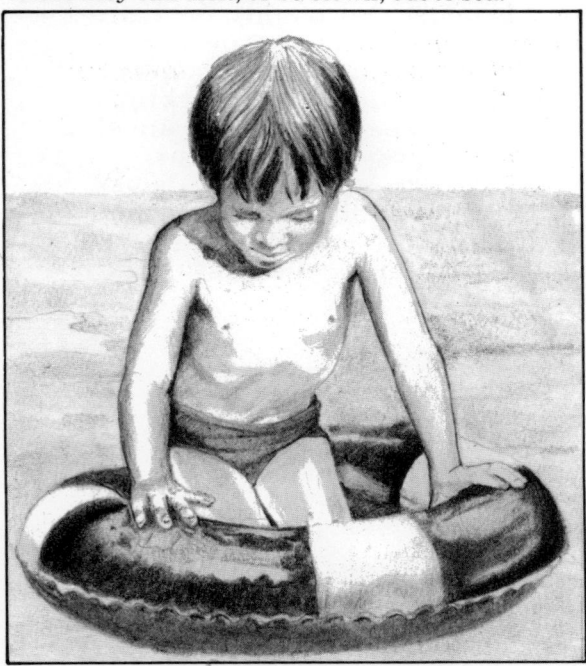

Ideally everyone out boating should be able to swim well, but even so, all should wear buoyancy vests, or better still life-jackets, at all times. Even on a hot sunny day, the water temperature may be bitterly cold and will rapidly sap the energy of even the strongest swimmer. Unless you are an experienced sailor, never take out a boat without an experienced colleague to teach you. Sailing requires skill and a thorough understanding of the craft, the sea and the weather.

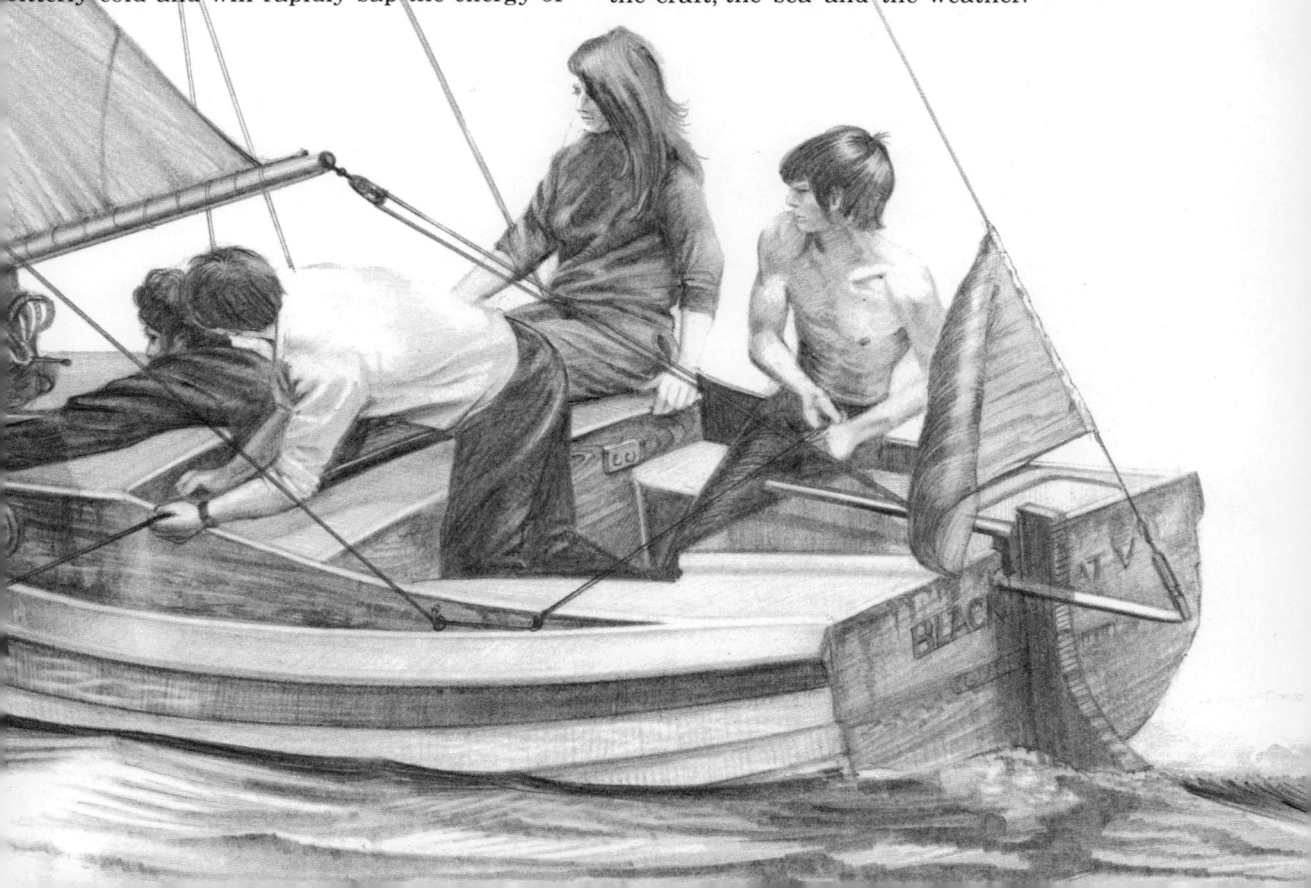

ALWAYS
- Prepare thoroughly for winter sports. Physical fitness is the best safeguard against accident
- Wear the approved clothing
- Take expert advice in choosing and adjusting equipment
- Listen to local advice about weather and snow conditions
- Stay on the marked 'piste' unless an experienced mountain skier

NEVER
- Wander off alone in unfamiliar mountain country
- Attempt to do more than you are capable of doing safely
- Ignore warning signs
- Remain at high altitude if you feel the effects of altitude sickness coming on
- Allow children on steep or long slopes unless they are proficient

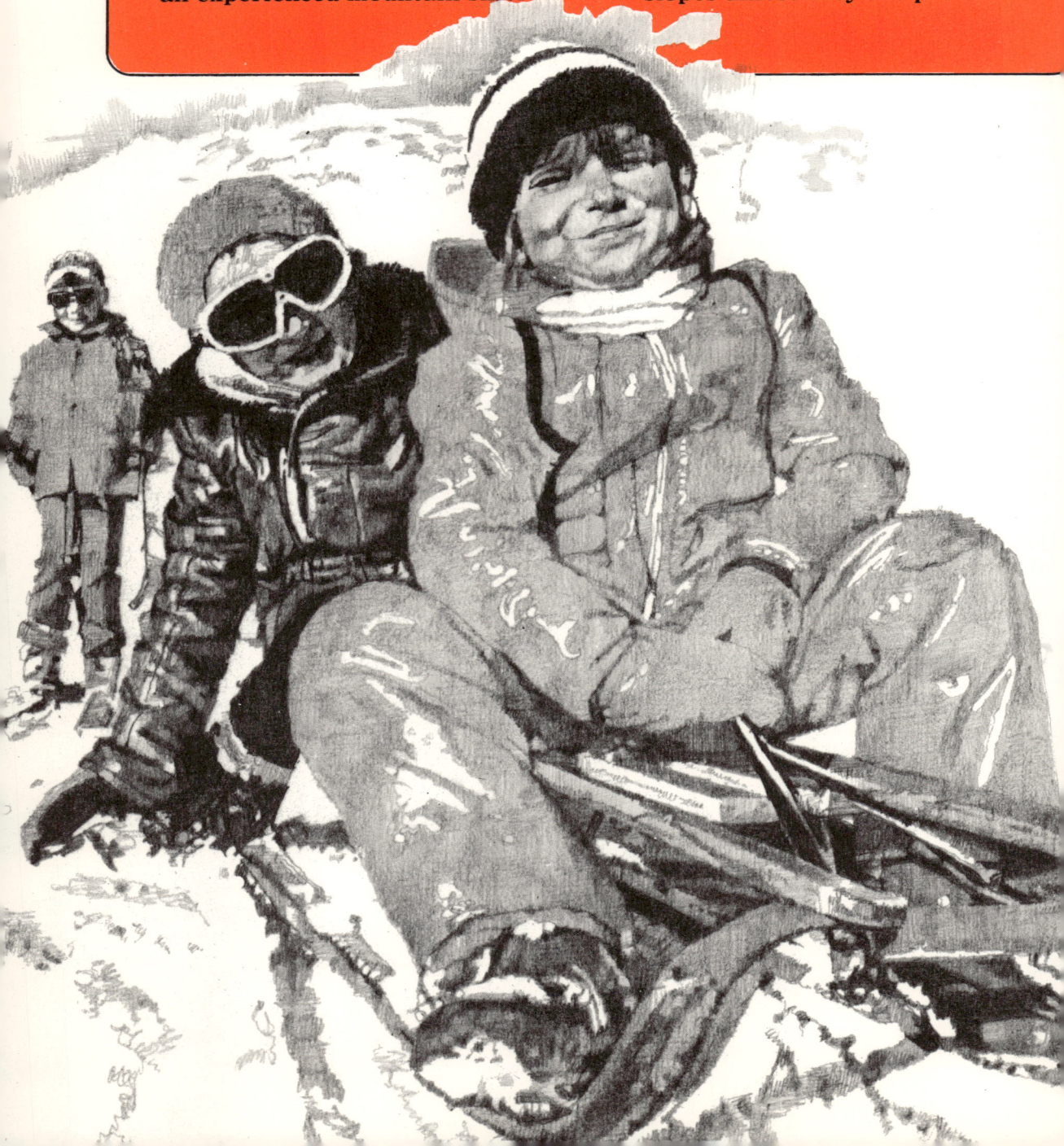

Winter Sports

If you are eager to take up the thrilling sport of skiing, but discouraged by tales of injury and danger, don't be put off. The vast majority of skiers do not suffer any injury – and sensible precautions can greatly reduce the potential hazards. Beginners are naturally at the greatest risk and should therefore take the elementary precaution of preparing thoroughly and having the correct equipment, properly fitted.

Skiing is extremely strenuous and the fitter you are, the less likely you are to have an accident. Start preparing at least a month before you go. Do the recommended pre-ski exercises and do as much walking and cycling as possible to strengthen the leg muscles. If possible, take lessons on a dry ski slope, or mogul (moving) slope.

Even with preparation, do not attempt too much during the first few days. A tired and stiff skier is at far greater risk than one who is relaxed and fit. More accidents happen in the late afternoon, when skiers are tired, than at any other time.

Not-so-fit beginners, and anyone who is not particularly athletic, should use the shorter type of ski, for the longer the ski, the faster you will travel and the more difficult it is to turn. Take expert advice in all matters of choosing and fitting equipment. The most important item is the boot; the weight and fitting should be absolutely right for the individual. Safety bindings hold the boot firmly on the ski but snap open in the event of a fall, protecting the leg from a severe wrench or even break. The bindings should be fitted and adjusted by an expert but always check the release *before* venturing onto the slope.

Skis are attached to the boots by straps to stop them shooting away in the event of a fall – a precaution against injury to skiers further down the slope and a great time-saver as hours can be wasted searching for a lost ski. However, injuries can be caused by the flailing skis of a falling skier and instead of the straps, many skiers now opt for 'ski-stoppers' – prongs lying flat along the top of the ski which snap open as the safety binding opens. They are effective in most conditions but are not suitable for use in deep powder snow.

Always wear at least two layers of insulating clothing under your ski suit. Do not be misled by bright sunshine and blue skies; temperatures on the mountain may be well below zero. Have a good meal before you set out otherwise tiredness and hunger will set in during the day. Beware too of altitude sickness. If you feel at all ill or light-headed, drop further down-slope immediately and stay at lower altitude for the day. Behavior on the slopes is of paramount importance. Always look round carefully before setting off; make allowance for less experienced skiers and do not approach corners too fast. Late in the season make allowance for variable snow conditions; hitting grass or a projecting rock at speed can have disastrous results.

Beware of the possibility of frostbite. This can be caused just as much by a strong wind as by intense cold, since each removes heat from the body. Therefore, when you are planning to go skiing, pay attention not only to the temperature, but also to the strength of the wind – most weather reports give wind-chill factors. If you notice that the skin of your face or hands is becoming numb and looks gray rather than pink, you should immediately go indoors or wrap the area with a dry covering. *Do not* rub the affected area with snow. If the frostbitten area has not improved after 15–30 minutes indoors, seek help from the ski patrol or a doctor. Rapid rewarming of the affected part is standard treatment for frostbite now, but should only be carried out by an experienced person. If hot water is used for this purpose, it should not be hotter than 104 degrees Fahrenheit.

Finally, a skiing party should always remain together matching their speed to that of the slowest member. This is particularly important when skiing away from the 'piste'. It is all too easy to lose your way when totally surrounded by snow and ever-changing slopes, and mists can come down with surprising speed in mountain country.

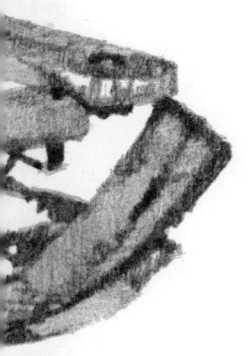

Sound preparation, correctly-fitted equipment, and common sense are the keys to the safe enjoyment of all winter sports.

Shooting

Modern guns for game shooting are powerful, accurate – and deadly. They need to be handled with the greatest possible care. Yet all too often these lethal weapons kill or maim not the animals and birds which are their targets but the hunters themselves, their companions or innocent passers-by.

Anyone handling a gun, or out on a shoot, for the first time will undoubtedly be aware of the potential dangers and seek to learn the fundamental rules for safety. Unfortunately, familiarity with guns and the hunting scene frequently breeds a casualness and a carelessness which all too easily leads to tragedy. The safety rules need not only to be learned: they must become so deeply ingrained that their practice is second nature.

Safety at all times
At any time when handling a gun it is always safest to assume that it is loaded, even if you have taken out the bullets or cartridges yourself. Never, *ever* point it at anyone, and always carry it safely, either in the crook of the arm with the barrels pointing towards the ground, or over the shoulder with the triggers upwards and the barrels pointing to the sky.

The barrels should be kept pointing in a safe direction even during the loading operation. For a breech-loading shotgun, for example, the gun should be closed by bringing the stock upwards–not the barrels. When clambering through, or climbing over, any obstacle the gun should always be unloaded, as it should be before it is picked up or put down, taken from someone else, put into a car or carried into the house.

Over the last century or so gun and cartridge design has evolved to produce a weapon that is safe, in the sense that it will not blow up in the hunter's face. But obstructions in the barrel can lead to serious accidents. So when the gun is taken out of its case, and before each loading while out in the field, look down the breech to ensure that there are no obstructions. Mud and snow can cause blockages, as can loading a shotgun with the wrong size cartridge: a 20-caliber cartridge, for instance, may drop unnoticed in a 12-caliber barrel; when the right size cartridge is loaded, the barrel could burst on firing with disastrous results.

The safety catch, which locks the triggers, should be kept ON until the gun is being raised to the shoulder to fire and it should be returned to the 'safe' position immediately after firing. The same general rules apply equally to rifled fire arms.

Precautions in the field
When out in the field, special care must be taken to ensure that no one comes into the line of fire of the shooter. Each huntsman should be aware of his 'safety zones,' the areas into which he can fire without endangering anyone. He should never, for example, swing his gun round, following a quarry, to such an angle as to bring his companions into his sights. When rough-shooting, guns should stay abreast of each other, particularly when a hedge or line of trees separates the hunters. Finally a gun must never be fired where you cannot see: beaters, farm workers, picnickers and even courting couples may be hidden behind trees or undergrowth.

Action
Gunshot wounds are often characterized by a small entry hole and a large exit wound with associated HEAVY BLEEDING (ACTION DETAILS pp. 62-69) and SHOCK (ACTION DETAILS pp. 90-91).

☎ *Get to a telephone as fast as possible and summon expert aid*

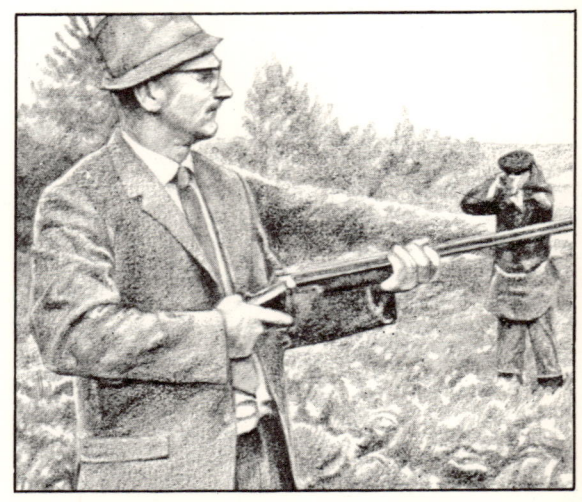

Potential disaster: the shooter, concentrating solely on his target, has swung too far, bringing a companion directly into his line of fire.

Racquet Sports and Jogging

Anyone taking up a strenuous sport after a number of years of relatively easy living should do so with care and with common sense, starting off with limited periods of light exercise and only gradually building up the length of time played and the degree of effort expended as the body becomes accustomed to the stresses imposed. A fast game of squash will raise the heartbeat from its normal 70 to 80 beats a minute to 120 or more within a few minutes; perfectly acceptable to a healthy body but a dangerous load to impose on the heart of a man carrying too much weight. Muscles and tendons may also suffer quite serious damage if the player fails to warm up properly before the game. All racquet sports involve bursts of acceleration and sudden stopping, starting and turning movements. If the body is well prepared there is little real danger of injury but if the muscles have not been limbered up the results can be torn achilles tendons or sprained knee joints.

Care and good sense on the court are also of great importance. A blow in the face from a racquet can be very serious and in many sports clubs and complexes, beginners are strongly advised to wear protective glasses.

Jogging and Running

Another activity currently enjoying great popularity is that of jogging and once again common sense is the key to safety. Even if in good physical condition, people over 40 should have a careful examination by their physician before setting out on the road, and all runners should begin slowly, increasing the amount of exercise as fitness improves.

Attention should be paid to footwear and to the surfaces on which you choose to run. An overweight man running on asphalt roads is very prone to stress fractures of the bones of the feet and lower legs. Well-fitting cushioned shoes are essential and it is wise, where possible, to select a course over parkland, a beach or the perimeter of a golf course.

In winter, the runner on open roads should take the precaution of wearing light-colored clothing, so that he is easily seen by drivers, and should always carry a sweater or tracksuit top to put on *as soon as he slows down*. Conversely, in the warm summer months, he should beware of the danger of heat exhaustion (**see pp 106-107**).

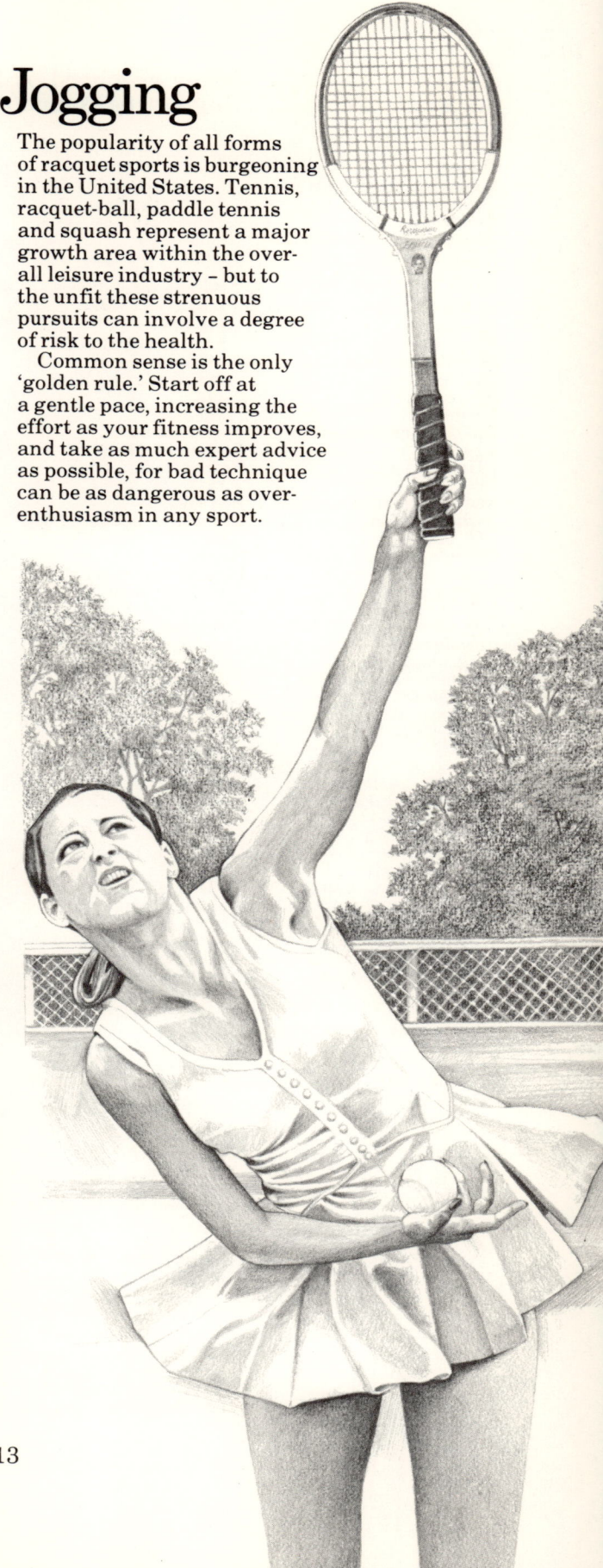

The popularity of all forms of racquet sports is burgeoning in the United States. Tennis, racquet-ball, paddle tennis and squash represent a major growth area within the overall leisure industry – but to the unfit these strenuous pursuits can involve a degree of risk to the health.

Common sense is the only 'golden rule.' Start off at a gentle pace, increasing the effort as your fitness improves, and take as much expert advice as possible, for bad technique can be as dangerous as over-enthusiasm in any sport.

Index

Index prepared by Brenda Hall MA,
Registered Indexer of the Society of Indexers

A

Abdominal emergencies, shock caused by, 90
Accidents
 first aid aims, action, 10-11, 48-9
 value of information, 49, 88-9, 101
 see also Road accidents
Acetaminophen, 44-5
Adhesive plasters, 43, 44-5, 68
Afterbirth, 93
Alcohol
 avoidance of excess, 18, 19
 Hazards, 12, 24-5, 63, 90, 91
 safe storage, 35
 when to withold, 61, 63, 90, 91
Altitude sickness, 111-12
Analgesics, 43, 44-5
Angina pectoris, 60-1
Ankles
 sprained, 84-5
 swollen, 99
Antacids, 44, 45
Antibacterial cream, 45
Antiseptics
 hazards, 63
 uses, 42-3, 44-5, 63, 96
Anxiety, significance of, 90
Appendix, perforated, shock caused by, 90
Arms
 broken, 72, 73
 cut, lacerated, 64-5
Artificial respiration
 following poisoning, 88
 in heart attack, 61
 methods, 50-7
 priorities, 10
 with heart massage, 51, 59
Asphyxia, unconsciousness due to, 70
Aspirin, 43, 44-5
Automobile accidents *see* Road Accidents

B

Babies
 accidents to, 12
 burns and scalds, 86
 care of new born, 93
 choking, action, 54
 heart massage, 59
Back troubles, 12, 16, 17, 18, 19, 39
Bandaging, bandages
 arm and hand, 64-5
 broken collarbone, 80-1
 broken jaw, 82-3
 broken limbs, 73, 74-5, 76-7
 burns and scalds, 87
 damaged pelvis, 79
 damaged spine, 78-9
 elbows, 67
 eyes, 94
 feet, 66-7
 fingers, 68-9
 following severe bleeding, 62
 head injuries, 69, 83
 improvised, 49
 in first aid kits, 42-3, 44
 knees, 66
 sprains, 84-5
Bath mats, 26, 30, 31
Bathroom hazards, 12-13, 26, 30, 31
Bedbugs, 96
Bedroom hazards, 12-13, 33
Bee stings, 96
Bladder injury, with broken pelvis, 79
Bleeding
 arm and hand, 64-5
 checking for, 70
 elbow, 66
 from fingers, 68
 from gunshot wounds, 112
 from head injuries, 69
 from puncture wounds, 66-7
 internal, 63, 72
 in urine, significance, 22
 knees, 66
 severe, action, priorities, 10, 49, 62, 63, 72, 78, 82, 83, 100-1
 slight, treatment, 63
 types of wound, 62
 see also Blood
Blood
 coughed up, significance of, 22, 63
 effects of sight of, 62, 91
 see also Plasma
Boils, 44
Bones, broken
 action, priorities, 49, 72, 100-1
 causes, types, 72
 checking for, 70, 71
 in children, 22
 shock caused by, 90
 vulnerability to, 12, 26-7
 with dislocation, 85
 see also individual bones
Bonfires, 38-9
Brachial pressure point, 63
Brake fluid, 36
Breastbone, fracture, 81
Breathing difficulties, 50, 60, 63, 90
 stopped, action, priorities, 10, 49, 50-1, 52-7, 61, 70, 72, 78, 82, 83, 100-1
 stopped, in poisoning, 88
 Stopped, while unconscious, 70
Bruising, bruises, significance of, 63
 treating, in children, 22
 vulnerability to, 12
Burns and scalds
 action, priorities, 15, 46, 47, 49, 86-7, 100-1
 causes, prevention, 16, 17
 shock caused by, 90
 vulnerability to, 12, 26
 what *not* to do, 86

C

Calamine lotion, 43, 45, 96, 97, 106, 108
Calf, cramp in, 84
Carpets, hazards from, 35
Camping safety, 102-3
Caving safety, 104-5
Casualties
 reassurance of, 10, 11, 49, 62, 72, 76, 97
 when, how to move, 10, 11, 49, 55, 70, 72, 74, 78-9, 101
Chemicals
 burns caused by, 87
 removal from danger, 49
 safe use, storage of, 14, 15, 20-1, 28, 29, 36-7, 38-9, 89
 swallowing corrosive, 50
Chest
 crushing of, 50
 wounds, open, action, 81
Childbirth
 management, 92-3
 signs of imminent, 92
Children
 accidents to, 12
 action for choking, 54
 burns and scalds, 86
 dangers from fire, 46
 giving artificial respiration, 53
 greenstick fractures, 72
 heart massage, 59
 poisoning, 11
 safety for, 14-15, 22-3, 28, 29, 30, 31, 36, 38-9, 100, 108-9, 113
 see also Alcohol, Chemicals, Drugs
Choking
 action, 10, 49, 54
 avoidance of, 50
Clothing
 for hikers, 104-5
 for skiing, 110-11
 safe airing of, 35
Cold (patient), significance of, 63
Cold, common, 44
Cold compresses, 84, 96
Collarbone, broken, 80-1
Compound fractures, 72
Concussion, 12, 70-1
Consciousness, clouded, significance of, 90
 see also Unconsciousness
Constipation, relief of, 45
Contractions, in childbirth, 92-3
Cooking
 for campers, 102
 safety during, 12, 16, 17, 20-1, 26, 28-9
Coronary thrombosis, 60-1; *see also* Heart attack
Corrosive liquids
 burns from, 87
 poisoning from, 88
 see also Chemicals
Cotton, 42-3, 44-5
Cramp, 84, 108
Crowd incidents, injuries following, 50, 81
Cuts
 treating, 18, 22, 68-9
 vulnerability to, 12, 15, 16, 17, 18, 26, 35, 64
 see also Bleeding
Cycling, safe, 22-3

D

Deficiency illness, 26
Diabetes, unconsciousness due to, 70
Diarrhea
 continual, cause of shock, 90
 hygiene measures, 44
 medicines, 44, 45
 on holiday, 99
Dislocations
 symptoms, action, 85
 vulnerability to, 12
 with fractures, 85
Distress Signals, International Alpine, 105
Dizziness *see* Giddiness
Dog bites, 97
Dressings
 following severe bleeding, 62
 for burns, scalds, 87
 for elbows, 67
 for fingers, 68
 for hands, arms, 64-5
 for head injuries, 69
 for knees, 66
 for puncture wounds, 66-

for slight injuries, 63
improvised, 49, 87
in first aid kits, 42-3 44-5
Drink, drinking
necessary after diarrhea, 44
to avoid sunstroke, 107
when to administer, withhold, 49, 61, 63, 71, 86, 88, 90
see also Alcohol
Driving, drivers
care with drugs, 43
safety for, 24, 25, 100
see also Road accidents
Driveway hazards, 12-13
Drowning, action following, 51, 54, 56-7
Drugs
hazard to elderly, 12, 20-1
overdose, breathing stopped by, 50
safe storage, 14-15, 20-1, 30-1, 32
teenage problems, 24-5
when to withhold, 61

E

Earache, relief of, 44
Ears, bleeding from, significance of, 63, 83
Elbow
bandaging, 67
broken, 72, 73
dislocated, 85
Elderly, hazards for, 12, 26-7, 32, 46
Electric blankets, 32
Electric equipment
extinguishing fires caused by, 46-7
safe use of, 15, 16, 17, 28-9, 30-1, 33, 34-5, 36-7, 39
see also Tools
Electric plugs, 16, 34, 35
Electric shocks
action, priorities, 56-7
breathing stopped by, 50
vulnerability to, 12
Emotional disturbance, effects of; 90, 91
Epilepsy,
unconsciousness due to, 70
Excitement, heart attack caused by, 60
Exercise, sound basis for, 18, 19
Exposure, dangers from, 105
Eye baths, 43, 44
Eyes
bandaging, 94
causes of injury, 39
damage by corrosive, 89
dilated pupils, significance of, 58, 59
protection, 36-7
Eyesight, defective, 26-7, 31

F

Faintness, fainting
action, 91
significance of, 63, 90, 91
Falls, 12, 15, 16, 17, 20-1, 26-7, 28, 29, 30-1, 32, 35
Family, accident causes, rates, 12
Fat see Cooking, Fire
Fats, animal, 19
Father, safety for, 18-19; see also Garage, Garden, Workshop
Feces, blood in, significance of, 22
Feet
broken, damaged, 77
cramp in, 84
danger from weaver fish, 108
puncture wounds, 66-7
swollen, 99
Femoral pressure point, 63
Filter masks, 36-7
Fingers
dislocation, 85
injuries, action, 68-9
Fire, fire hazards
action for victim of, 55
clothing, 46, 47
extinguishers, 28, 46-7
guards, 20-1, 26-7
incidence, 12
procedures, 46, 47
safety measures, 15, 16, 17, 28, 29, 35, 46 102-3
withdrawal from danger, 10, 49
Fireplaces, safe use of, 35
First aid
aims, priorities, 10-11 48-9
kits, 42-3, 44-5
value of information, 49, 88-9, 101
Fish hook, removal of, 95
Flea bites, 96
Floors, slippery, 16, 26 28, 29, 30, 31, 35
Food
avoidance of excess, 19
poisoning, 99
when to withhold, 63, 71
Fractures, types, 72; see also Bones, broken, and individual bones
Frayed cables, 16
Frostbite, 111

G

Garages, hazards, safety in, 12-13, 18, 36-7, 68
Gardens
hazards, safety in, 12, 14-15, 20-1, 68
poisonous plants, 40-1
Gas, gas appliances
action for victim of, 10, 50, 55
hazards, safe use of, 12, 28, 31, 102
removal from danger, 49
Gauze (sterile)
for burns, scalds, 87
in first aid kits, 42-3, 44-5
Gauze bandages, 67, 68-9
Giddiness
significance of, 63, 90, 91, 106
vulnerability to, 26-7
Glyceryl trinitate, 61
Gnat bites, 96
Grazes, 22
Greenstick fractures, 72; see also Bones, broken, and individual bones
Guns, safe use of, 112

H

Hallways, hazards of, 12-13
Hands
broken, 73
cramp, 84
incised wounds, 64-5
Handicapped people, vulnerability of, 12
Handrails, 26, 30-1, 32
Headache, significance of, 105
Head injuries
bandaging, 69
unconsciousness due to, 70
Heart
stopped, action priorities, 49, 58-9 100-1
stopped, signs, symptoms, 58
structure, functions, 58
Heart attack
action, 60-1
causes, 39
defined, 60
shock caused by, 90
signs, symptoms, 60, 61
unconsciousness due to, 70
vulnerability to, 19
Heart compression,
massage use of, 52, 54 58, 59, 61
with artificial respiration, 51, 56, 57, 59
Heaters
bathroom, 30-1
fireguard protection, 35
for trailers, 102
open, portable, safe use of, 16, 17, 20-1, 32
Heat exhaustion, 106
Heatstroke, 106
Heimlich Method, 51
High voltage electric shock, 58
Hiking, safety in, 104-5
Holger-Nielsen artificial respiration, 54-5, 56-7
Home accidents, rates, 12
Home cures, 44-5
Horsefly bites, 96
Household maintenance, hazards of, 12
Hygiene
following diarrhea, 44
with pets, 20-1
Hypothermia, 26, 105

I

Immunizations, 99
Indigestion medicines, 43, 44, 45
Infants see Babies
Infection, danger following burns, 86, 87
Inhalation injuries, 12
Injuries, internal
signs, symptoms, 10, 22
to chest cavity, 81
with broken bones, 72, 79
Insect bites, stings, 42, 43, 45, 50, 96
Insurance, for travellers, 99
Internal bleeding see Bleeding
Internal injuries see Injuries
International Alpine Distress Signal, 105

J

Jaw
broken, 82-3
dislocated, 85
Jellyfish stings, 97, 108
Jet lag, 99
Jogging, 113

K

Kerosene camping stove 102; see also Heaters
Kiss of life see Mouth to Mouth artificial respiration
Kitchen, hazards, safety in, 12-13, 16-17, 28-9

115

Knees
  bandaging, 66
  broken kneecap, 76
  sprained, 84-5
Knives, safe use, storage of, 15, 16, 17, 20-1, 28

L

Labor, stages of, 92-3
Ladders, safe use of, 14-15, 16, 18-19
Lavatory, hazards, 12-13, 26
Laxatives, 45
Leeches, 96
Legs, broken, 74-5
Lemon juice, for wasp stings, 96
Lethargy, significance of, 105
Lice, 96
Life jackets, 108
Lifting see Weights
Lips,
  blueness, significance of, 60
  moistening a conscious burned casualty's, 11
Living room, hazards, safety in, 12-13, 34-5
Lungs
  danger from broken ribs, 81
  protective masks, 36, 37
  structure, function, 58

M

Malaria, immunization 99
Mats, non-slip, 26, 30, 31
Medicines, home, 44-5; see also Drugs
Methanol for jellyfish stings, 108
Mosquito bites, 96
Mother, safety for, 16-17, 28-9
Mouth, sting inside, 96
Mouth to mouth artificial respiration, 52-3, 54-5, 56-7, 88, 93

N

Nausea, significance of, 90, 105
Neck, checking for injury, 10
Nose
  bleeding from, significance of, 44, 63, 83
  protection with mask, 36, 37

O

Over-exertion, heart attack caused by, 39, 60
Oxygen, body needs, 51

P

Pain
  abdominal, significance of, 22
  fainting caused by, 91
  severe, significance of, 60
Pain killers, 43, 44-5
Paints, safe use of, 36-7
Parents, attitudes to teenagers, 24-5
Pedestrians, road safety for, 100
Pelvis, broken, 79
Perspiration, significance of, 91; see also Sweating
Pesticides see Chemicals
Pets
  and hygiene, 20-1
  bites, scratches from, 97
  safety for, 39
Pillow, suffocation by, 50
Plants
  poisonous, 40-1
  stings from, 97
Plasma, shock caused by loss of, 90
Plastic bags, dangers of, 12, 20-1, 28, 50
Poisoning, poisons
  action, priorities, 40, 88
  breathing stopped by, 50
  from garden plants, 40-1
  unconsciousness due to, 70
  vulnerability to, 12
  see also Chemicals, Drugs
Poliomyelitis
  damage to breathing mechanism from, 50
  immunization, 99
Ponds, garden, 14-15,
Pregnancy and vacations, 99
Pressure direct, 62
Pressure points, 63
Pulse, significance of abnormal, 58, 59, 63, 90, 106

R

Rabies, 97
Racquet sports, 19, 113
Reassurance, importance for casualty, 10, 11, 49, 62, 72, 86, 97
Recovery position, 10, 50, 53, 70-1, 88, 91
Red Cross Society, 10
Respiratory system, structure, functions, 50, 51
Ribs, broken, 81
Road accidents
  avoidance, 24, 25, 43, 100
  breathing stopped following, 50
  first aid action, 100-1
  frequency, 12
  injuries to chest, 81
  priority action, 100
  value of information, 49, 88-9, 101

S

Safety pins, 43
Sailing, safety in, 109
Salt deficiency, 84, 106
Sandflies, 96
Scalds, scalding
  of the throat, 50
  shock caused by, 90
  vulnerability to, 31
  see also Burns and scalds
Scissors, 43
Scorpion stings, 96
Sea urchins, 108
Shellfish, 99
Shock
  action, 46, 47, 49, 71, 72, 82, 90, 91
  defined, 90
  conditions causing, 62, 74, 81, 90, 96, 112
  following road accident, 101
  heart attack caused by, 60
  signs, symptoms, 90
  unconsciousness due to, 70
Shooting, safety during, 112-13
Shoulder, dislocated, 85
Shower units, 31
Sickness see Vomiting
Sighing, significance of, 63
Simple fractures, 72; see also Bones, broken, and under individual bones
Skateboarding, safety in, 22, 23
Skiing, safety in, 110-11
Skin
  blue-gray, significance of, 58, 59
  clammy, significance of, 63, 90
  hot dry, significance of, 106
  pale, significance of, 58, 59, 60, 90, 91
Skull, fractured, 83
Slings, 49, 73
Slipped disk, 16
Smallpox vaccination, 99
Smoke, action for victim of, 50, 55
Smoking, hazards of, 12, 18, 19, 24
Snake bites, 97
Sodium bicarbonate paste, for bites, stings, 96
Speech, slurred, significance of, 105
Spelunking, 104-5
Spiders, poisonous, 96
Spine, injuries to
  action, 78-9, 101
  breathing stopped by, 50
  checking for, 10
Splinters, wood, 12, 22, 95
Splints, 73, 74-5, 76-7
Sport, hazards of, 24, 25
Sprains, 12, 66, 84-5
Stairs, hazards, safe use, 12-13, 16, 20-1, 26-7, 32
Steps, step-ladders, hazards, safe use, 14-15, 16, 18-19
Sternum, fracture of, 81
Stomach emergencies, shock caused by, 90
Stove Top, 17
Strains, 12, 85
Stroke, unconsciousness due to, 70
Strangulation, 50
Stretcher, lifting on to, 78-9
Suffocation
  breathing stopped by, 50
  from plastic bags, 12, 20-1, 28, 50
  vulnerability to, 12
  while unconscious, 70
Sunburn, 43, 45, 106
Sunstroke, 91, 106-7
Swabs, sterile, 44-5
Swaying, significance of, 91
Sweating, significance of, 60, 90
Swimming
  cramp during, 108
  need for instruction in, 24
Sylvester method of artificial respiration, 56-7

T

Teenagers, hazards for, 12, 24-5
Television sets, safe use of, 19, 35
Temperature, raised, significance of, 106
Tennis, 19, 113
Tetanus
  danger of infection, 97
  immunization, 99
Thighs
  broken, 74-5
  cramp in, 84
Thirst, significance of, 63, 90; see also Drink
Thorns, removal of, 95
Three-year old children, hazards, safety for, 20-1
Throat, effect of damage to, 50
Throttling, 50
Ticks, 90, 96
Toenails, 26
Tongue, obstruction caused by, 50

Tools, safe use, storage of, 14-15, 18-19, 20-1, 36-7, 38-9
Toothache, 44
Toxic liquids, withdrawal from danger, 10; *see also* Chemicals
Trachea, blockage, compression of, 50, 51
Trailer safety, 102-3
Travel sickness, 43, 45
Tree-climbing, 22
Tweezers, 43
Typhoid fever immunization, 99

U

Umbilical cord, 93
Unconsciousness
 action, 10, 49, 70-1, 101
 causes, 70, 88

Urine, blood in, significance of, 22

V

Vacations
 food hygiene, 99
 immunizations, 99
 insurance, 99
Vapours, inflammable, 36
Ventilation
 of poisonous fumes, 36
Vinegar, for wasp stings, 96
Vision, impaired, significance of, 90, 105; *see also* Eyesight
Vomiting
 continual, shock caused by, 90
 medicines, 44, 45
 significance, 50, 90, 106

W

Wasp stings, 96
Water
 drinking, sterilization of, 99
 fire extinguishers, 46, 47
 when to administer, withhold, 44, 49, 61, 63, 71, 86, 88, 90
Water-skiing, 109
Water sports, safety in, 108-9
Weaver fish, 108
Weights, lifting, carrying, 12, 16, 17, 18, 19
Windows, safe use of, 20-1, 33
Windpipe, blockage, compression of, 50, 51
Winter sports, safety in, 110-11

Workshops, safety in, 18, 36-7, 68; *see also* Tools
Wounds
 action, 18, 22, 64-5, 66-7, 97, 112
 avoiding infection, 18, 19
 contused, 62
 gunshot, 112
 incised, 62, 64-5
 lacerated, 62, *see also* Cuts
 presenting dressings sticking, 63
 puncture, 12, 62, 66-7, 97
Wrist, sprained, 84-5

Y

Yellow fever, immunization, 99

Acknowledgments

Many organizations and individuals have given invaluable help in the preparation of this book. The publishers wish to extend their thanks to them all, and in particular to the following.

The Royal Society for the Prevention of Accidents; The British Red Cross Society; The Health Education Council; The Department of Prices and Consumer Protection; The Pharmaceutical Society; MK Electric Limited; The Fire Protection Association; The British Standards Institution; Chubb Fire Security Limited; Neighbours (of Kingsbury) Limited; The Flowers and Plants Council; British Museum (Natural History); HAES Systems; Wolseley Webb Limited; Flymo Limited; Camping Club of Great Britain and Ireland; British Mountaineering Council; National Caving Association; British Field Sports Society; Ski Club of Great Britain.

Our special thanks to Mr J F G Coles, Secretary-Association of the St. John Ambulance Association and Brigade, for help and advice and for checking the page-proofs; and to 'Wallie', Pat, Joan and Gilbert of Casualties Union for their enormous contribution in demonstrating the techniques described in *Accident Action*.

Illustrations throughout the *Action* pages of the book were drawn from photographs taken by David Messer.

Artists' Credits

Our thanks to the following artists whose work appears in *Accident Action*.

Clare Davies (Artist Partners), pp 13, 16/17, 18/19, 20/21, 22/23, 25, 26/27, 28/29, 30/31, 32/33, 34/35, 36/37, 38, 112
Carol Binch (Artist Partners), pp 102/103
Harry Hants (Artist Partners), pp 106/107
Cecil Vieweg (Artist Partners), pp 98, 110
Studio Briggs, inset p 34 and key-line preparation throughout the book
David and Sue Holmes, pp 6, 10/11, 46/47, 50/51, 52/53, 54/55, 56/57, 58/59, 60/61, 62/63, 64/65, 66/67, 68/69, 70/71, 72/73, 74/75, 76/77, 78/79, 80/81, 82/83, 84/85, 86/87, 88/89, 90/91, 92/93, 94/95, 96/97, 105
Keith Harmer, pp 14/15, 108
Andy Farmer, pp 40/41, 100/101, 104, 107, 109, 113

Editor	Martyn Bramwell
Art Director	Nicholas Eddison
Assistant Editor	Pendleton Campbell
Research Assistant	Jane Butcher
Designer	Clare Judd
Assistant Designer	Doug Hewitt
Editorial Assistant	Sue Brown
Editorial Consultant	Victor Stevenson
Production	Kenneth Cowan

BREATHING STOPPED	**50/57**	Causes of breathing stoppages and the techniques of artificial respiration. Emergency action in cases of drowning, choking, electric shock and suffocation.
HEART STOPPED	**58/61**	Causes of cardiac arrest, and emergency life-saving action. The 'heart attack' – what it is and how to deal with it.
BLEEDING	**62/69**	The main types of wound and how they are caused. External and internal bleeding. Techniques of arresting heavy bleeding and of bandaging the casualty's wound.
LOSS OF CONSCIOUSNESS	**70/71**	Emergency action to be taken in all cases of unconsciousness. The recovery position and its importance in ensuring the safety of an accident victim.
BROKEN BONES	**72/83**	The types of break and the direct and indirect effects on the body. Techniques of bandaging and of immobilizing the injured part. How to move an injured person safely and securely.
SPRAIN, STRAIN AND DISLOCATION	**84/85**	Injuries to the muscles alone and to the muscles and tendons of the joints. The methods of bandaging, splinting and moving an injured person safely.